Southern Missionary College
Division Of Nursing, Library
711 Lake Estelle Drive
Orlando, Florida 32803

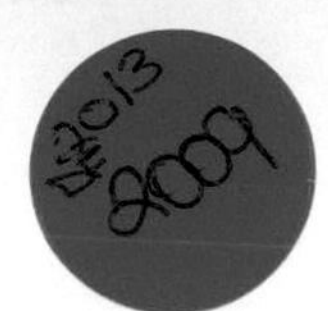

DIABETIC CARE
IN
PICTURES

Seminole Community College
Division Of Health Library
711 Lake Estelle Drive
Orlando, Florida 32803

DIABETIC CARE IN PICTURES

Simplified Statements with Illustrations Prepared for the Use of the Patient

Helen Rosenthal, B.S.
Former Director, Frances Stern Nutrition Center, New England Medical Center Hospitals
Former Assistant in Medicine at the School of Medicine, Tufts University

Joseph Rosenthal, M.D.
Assistant Professor of Medicine at the School of Medicine, Tufts University
Physician-in-Charge, Diabetes Clinic
Associate Staff (Internal Medicine)
New England Medical Center Hospitals

WK 810 .R815 1968

4th Edition

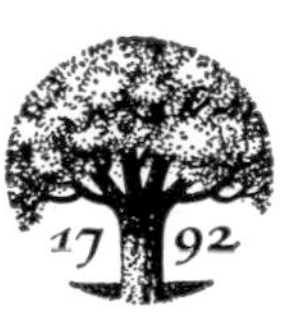

5427

J. B. LIPPINCOTT COMPANY
PHILADELPHIA and TORONTO

Southern Missionary College
Division Of Nursing, Library
711 Lake Estelle Drive
Orlando, Florida 32803

FOURTH EDITION

Copyright © 1968, by J. B. Lippincott Company

Copyright 1946, 1953, 1960, by J. B. Lippincott Company

This book is fully protected by copyright and, with the exception of brief extracts for review, no part of it may be reproduced in any form by print, photoprint, microfilm or any other means without the written permission of the publishers.

Distributed in Great Britain by
Pitman Medical Publishing Co., Limited, London

Library of Congress Card Number 68-20605
Printed in the United States of America

3 5 6 4 2

To J. S. R.

PREFACE

In 1946 the authors embarked on the first edition of DIABETIC CARE IN PICTURES. During the intervening years researchers and practitioners have continued to investigate diabetes and to improve treatment for the patient. The present edition has been written to keep pace with modern concepts. New editions, however, are written not only to update information but in response to the many invaluable suggestions which have resulted from successful use of the book by the physician and the professional worker as well as the patient. It is hoped that the reorganization of this book reflects a blending of the new and the old, thus giving the patient a convenient reference manual that will supplement and reinforce the doctor's prescription and provide a better understanding of his condition. Every attempt has been made to anticipate questions and to offer a workable regimen for the patient and his family.

The latest medical treatment for diabetes is presented and interpreted in this edition. As before, special attention is given to insulin preparations in current use and to the equipment available for their injection. Particular consideration is provided in the detailed discussion of the oral hypoglycemic agents. The newest and more rapid and convenient methods for testing urine are also included. In addition, the principles of physical and mental health, especially in their relation to total diabetic treatment, are emphasized.

The management of diabetes requires a knowledge of food values so that choices of foods can be made within the limitations of the diet prescription. Important as it is to have alternatives—or exchanges, as they are called—the wide variety of foods available may cause confusion. With this in mind, a revised compilation of food exchanges is presented, both verbally and graphically, in a manner that enables the patient to adapt his diet more easily to his particular needs. This edition utilizes the more recent analyses of foods and the exchange lists have been expanded to include many new food products found in today's market. The reader will be especially interested in the section on popular combination dishes. It is hoped that a practicable knowledge of the exchanges will facilitate decisions in food selection and allow the patient to "eat out" with ease and confidence. The patient who may have a coexistent condition requiring further modification of his diet will find sample diabetic diets adjusted to meet sodium restriction, a bland, a low residue and a liquid diet. A table of food values of commonly used foods, as well as a comprehensive glossary, appear in the appendix.

It has been the authors' experience, in private practice and in the Diabetes Clinic of the Tufts–New England Medical Center (Boston), that patients and their families can find help and encouragement through the additional information supplied by a simplified text. The fourth edition of DIABETIC CARE IN PICTURES is presented in the hope that it will fulfill these needs.

We wish to express our appreciation to those who have aided in the preparation of this edition: the patients who continue to prove the value of the teaching methods through their constant use and appraisal of the previous three editions; Mrs. Gertrude K. Soderstrom, B.S., M.Ed., former Staff Nutritionist, Frances Stern Nutrition Center, for meticulous care in the revision of material concerned with diet and food values; Mrs. Pearl C. Baker, B.S., M.Ed., former Staff Nutritionist, Frances Stern Nutrition Center, for generous time and valuable counsel; Eli Lilly and Company for continued interest and assistance; and the J. B. Lippincott Company, especially J. Brooks Stewart, Medical Editor, and J. Stuart Freeman, Jr., Production Editor.

Helen and Joseph Rosenthal

FOREWORD

As the fourth edition of DIABETIC CARE IN PICTURES becomes a reality, a sweeping backward glance to twenty-two years ago when the first edition of this book was published is a reminder not only of its usefulness but also of its impact on the practices of diabetic patients. This compilation of methods, materials and information, developed from many years of treating and teaching diabetic patients by the authors, has provided a means of sharing with many other patients and professional colleagues the success which the authors have achieved.

Encouraged and assisted by the late Frances Stern, who founded and directed the Nutrition Center which continues to bear her name, the authors have been able to extend the influence and application of the philosophy and teachings of the Diabetes Clinic and of the Frances Stern Nutrition Center far beyond the Tufts–New England Medical Center in Boston. As the Frances Stern Nutrition Center now marks the occasion of its golden anniversary, it seems appropriate to acknowledge the originality, and extensive application of the methods which have survived and grown in effectiveness during the past fifty years.

As far as can be determined, the food exchange system whereby foods of approximately equal nutrient content may be exchanged for one another was begun by Frances Stern in 1918 at the Boston Dispensary (now a part of the Tufts–New England Medical Center) as an aid in teaching diabetic patients of foreign birth who sought treatment at the Boston Dispensary's Diabetes and Food Clinics. The primary and original purpose of the food exchanges was to show foreign-born patients how their native foods could be used in the diabetic diet. Nine years later (1927), the first description of this method of patient education was published by Frances Stern and Jean Reyner in the Journal of the American Medical Association. A year later (1928), Miss Stern interested a talented young artist working at the U. S. Department of Agriculture in her idea of reproducing models of various size food servings in wax as a visual aid in teaching the food exchanges. Stimulated, encouraged and helped by Frances Stern, Mrs. Russell Roller of Washington embarked on the then new venture of creating wax food models. A few years later in the 1930's, "picture sheets" were developed as "take-home materials" for patients. These "picture sheets" effectively supplemented the individualized diets and the visualization of serving sizes which the wax food models demonstrated at the Clinic. After a decade of further development and use, the set of picture sheets for eleven nutrients was copyrighted, and in 1946 they were included in the first edition of DIABETIC CARE IN PICTURES. In the interim, it has become evident that the food exchange system is applicable in the teaching of *all* patients on any of the many other restricted diets! Thus, as society became increasingly cosmopolitan, the food exchange system has provided for adapting a restricted diet to seasons and holidays, as well as food preferences and likes and dislikes.

Since their beginning, the food exchanges have been revised, expanded and updated as new food products suitable for use on a restricted diet have appeared on the market, as methods for determining food composition have been developed and as new data on food composition have become available. The food exchanges and the picture sheets of this edition of DIABETIC CARE IN PICTURES have been revised, as has been the practice with each new edition.

Following the first edition of this book in 1946, a joint committee of the American Diabetes Association and the United States Public Health Service published in 1950 the Meal Planning Booklet, which also includes food exchanges. The reader will note that the food exchanges of the latter publication differ in some instances from the food exchanges of DIABETIC CARE IN PICTURES. These differences reflect the updating of this new edition and the hope that the patient will use a variety of the new foods and new food products. The authors believe that the continued revision and expansion of food exchanges will encourage patients to vary their diets. They further reason that the satisfied patient is more likely to live within the limitations of the *few* restrictions which *are* imposed by the diabetic diet.

The professional person using this book will find it a meaningful and logical approach to patient teaching as well as a helpful tool in assuring coordination and correlation of factual information. Whether the teaching is done by one or several professional persons, each one by being more knowledgeable of the total needs of the patient can be more effective. In many areas the nurse will assume the primary responsibility for total patient teaching. In other instances, it may be the dietitian who assumes this responsibility. But, to whomever this responsibility belongs, will come the challenge and satisfaction of comprehensive teaching.

Those of us who are privileged to have been students and colleagues of Dr. and Mrs. Joseph Rosenthal appreciate the meaningful and fortunate experience that has been ours. Through this book the reader—patient, family and professional person—may share the knowledge, human understanding and skill of the authors. The goals of this book have been stated by the authors in the Preface. May the reader achieve these goals and thereby experience some of the motivation which the dedication, enthusiasm and understanding of the authors have generated in their own patients, students and colleagues.

Baltimore, Maryland
April 10, 1968

Clare E. Forbes, B.S., M.P.H.
Chief, Division of Nutrition
Maryland Department of Health
Former Director, Frances Stern Nutrition Center.

CONTENTS

TO THE PATIENT

This book tells the story of diabetes and its treatment. The knowledge supplied will be a means of helping you to share with the physician the responsibility for the control of the disease. Constant use of the information in these pages should remove anxiety or fear and give you a feeling of security. Treatment will then become a routine part of your daily living, and you will be able to live a normal, happy life.

1. DIABETES* AND ITS TREATMENT

Diabetes* is not uncommon and occurs universally. Recent statistics† indicate that in the United States more than 2½ million persons are known to have diabetes. It is estimated that more than 1½ million have undetected diabetes, making a total of 4 million people with diabetes.‡

When the body is not able to use and store food in a normal fashion, diabetes follows. The exact cause is not fully understood, but it is generally agreed that there is involved an insufficient supply of insulin, improper utilization of insulin, or interference with the action of insulin in the body. For many years it was thought that the pancreas, from which insulin is derived, was the only gland related to diabetes. However, investigations have shown that other glands may be involved as well, and conditions associated with these glands may require treatment.

Insulin is a hormone normally manufactured in the body by the pancreas, a gland located just below and behind the stomach (Fig. 1). Within the pancreas are special clusters of cells called islands of Langerhans.§ Certain cells, namely, beta cells, within the islands of Langerhans, supply insulin which is released from the pancreas into the blood stream as it is needed for the proper use and storage of sugar which is derived from food.

The diagnosis of diabetes can be confirmed by definite laboratory tests of the blood and the urine. Although the exact nature of the cause of diabetes is not yet fully understood, years of research have yielded much knowledge concerning this disease and its treatment. While it must be stated that diabetes cannot be cured as of the present time, current investigations and improved methods of treatment point to promising possibilities for a more normal way of living and a longer span of life.

NORMAL USE AND STORAGE OF FOOD IN THE BODY

The many body functions and processes are regulated with astonishing detail of accuracy, and this holds true for the metabolism of sugar in the body. Normally, insulin supplies are adequate, and the body can use and store as much sugar as is derived from the food in the diet. The sugar is obtained not only from all of the carbohydrate in food (p. 10) but from

* Diabetes mellitus, the full name for this condition, is derived from Greek words meaning "flowing through" (diabetes) and "honey," or "sweets" (mellitus).

† Fact Sheet on Diabetes, American Diabetes Association, 1967.

‡ On the basis of an estimated total U.S. population of 200,000,000 as of July 31, 1967.

§ Named after the German scientist, Langerhans, who first called attention to these cells.

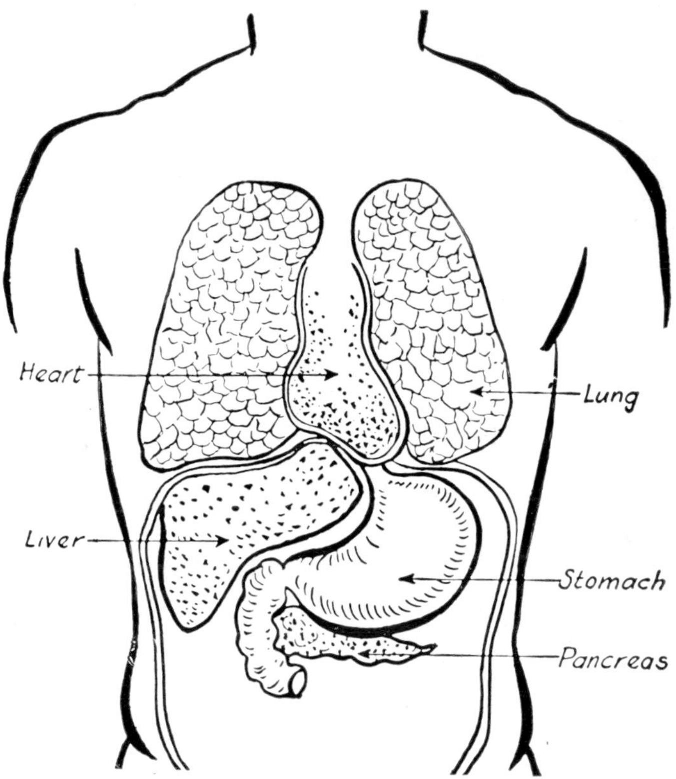

FIG. 1. Diagram showing position of pancreas in the body.

approximately 60% of the protein in the diet (p. 10); and from about 10% of the fat in the diet (p. 10).

In the normal processes of digestion the sugar derived from food is converted in the intestines into glucose. Then the glucose is taken up from the intestinal tract by the blood stream and carried to the liver where it is changed into still another form of sugar called glycogen. This glycogen is stored in the liver, the muscles and in other body tissues to become available whenever there is a demand for energy. As the need occurs, the glycogen is then reconverted into glucose, since it is in this form that sugars are utilized by the body.

Normally, with adequate amounts of available insulin, there is a wonderful regulatory mechanism in the body in regard to the utilization of sugar. When more food is furnished by the diet than is required for immediate use, this excess food is stored as available sugar, or it can be converted into fat and stored throughout the body as fat deposits. Sugar is car-

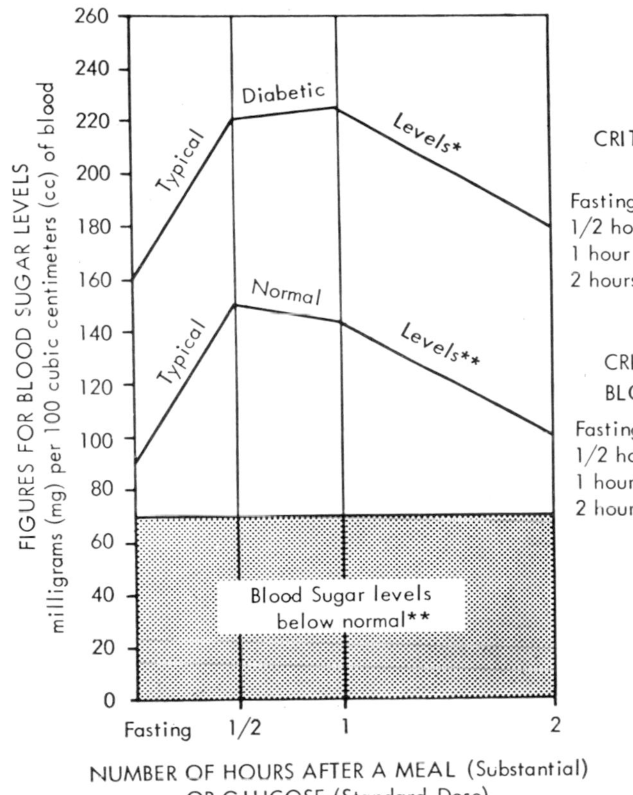

CRITERIA FOR DIAGNOSIS OF DIABETES

Fasting more than 110 mg/100 cc
1/2 hour more than 160 mg/100 cc
1 hour more than 160 mg/100 cc
2 hours more than 120 mg/100 cc

CRITERIA FOR NORMAL BLOOD-SUGAR-LEVELS

Fasting less than 100 mg/100 cc
1/2 hour less than 160 mg/100 cc
1 hour less than 160 mg/100 cc
2 hours less than 110 mg/100 cc

*Sugar present in the urine usually
**No sugar present in the urine usually

FIG. 2. Normal and diabetic blood-sugar levels. (Venous blood—true glucose method)

ried to the various parts of the body through the blood stream; therefore, a certain amount of sugar is present in the blood at all times to be used by the body for food and energy. However, when all the processes of normal sugar metabolism are taking place the amounts of sugar in the blood (blood-sugar-levels) remain within normal limits and no sugar is present in the urine at any time (Fig. 2).

DIABETES AND CARBOHYDRATE (SUGAR) METABOLISM

The normal use and storage of sugar does not take place when diabetes is present because there is insufficient utilizable insulin for sugar metabolism. Instead, the sugar derived from food accumulates in the blood stream, causing blood-sugar levels to rise beyond normal limits (Fig. 2). After certain limits have been reached, sugar is "spilled over" from the kidneys into the urine.

As a rule, most signs and symptoms commonly associated with diabetes are directly related to these increased amounts of sugar in the blood stream and to the presence of sugar in the urine.

SIGNS AND SYMPTOMS OF DIABETES

As previously stated, diabetes is usually recognized by the presence of sugar in the urine. In most instances this is accompanied by other typical signs and symptoms which may have developed either gradually or suddenly.

Among the earliest of these is the passing of large amounts of urine (*polyuria*) and frequency of urination. These result from the loss of body fluids used for the elimination of the excess amounts of sugar. When large quantities of fluids are excreted in the urine they need to be replaced in the body. This causes excessive thirst (*polydipsia*). Since much of the food consumed cannot be utilized, there is a loss of body weight as well as an increase of appetite (*polyphagia*) and hunger. Weakness and fatigue occur often because the sugar in the diet cannot be utilized for the body's energy requirement. Generalized or localized itching is frequent, especially in the genital region. Other manifestations include pain, numbness and tingling in the hands and the feet, disturbances in vision, as well as irritability and nervousness.

Since diabetes can be present without the characteristic signs and symptoms, a periodic medical examination should always include a routine urinalysis (urine examination) and a blood-sugar determination (one or two hours after a regular meal). When there is a history of diabetes in the family, especially in the obese person, a blood-sugar determination is definitely indicated. Many areas in the United States have Community Screening Programs for the detection of diabetes.

HEREDITY AND DIABETES

There is reliable scientific information, generally accepted by physicians and scientists, that a tendency toward diabetes may be inherited. In fact, it is often referred to as a hereditary disease. According to the Mendelian Law of Heredity, diabetes seems to be inherited as a recessive trait, meaning that it cannot be inherited from one side of the family alone (p. 183, Personal and Social Factors).

Figure 3 illustrates the relationship of heredity and expected incidence of diabetes according to the Mendelian Law of Heredity.

When there is a family history of diabetes, a physical examination each year is indicated. Also, there should be an earnest effort to maintain desirable or ideal weight, that is, the weight considered the best for the individual according to sex, age, height and body

HEREDITY AND EXPECTED INCIDENCE OF DIABETES*

How the Mendelian Law of Heredity Applies to Parents and Their Children

KEY

Nondiabetic

Diabetic

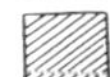

Diabetic Carrier

A carrier is an individual, male or female, who, although free of a disease, transmits to his or her offspring the tendency to, or the potentiality for, the disease from his or her ancestors.

When a diabetic marries a nondiabetic who is not a carrier, it is almost certain that none of their children will develop diabetes, but they will be carriers.

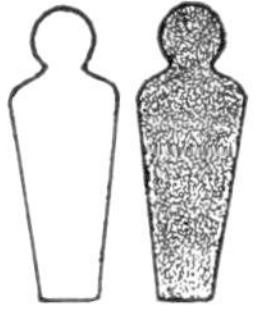

In a marriage of two carriers, 25% of their children will be diabetic; 75% will be carriers.

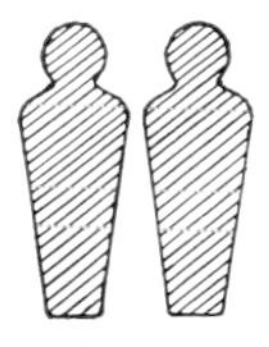

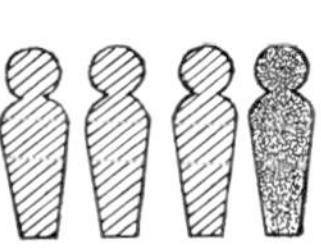

When a diabetic marries a carrier, 50% of their children will become diabetic, and 50% will be carriers.

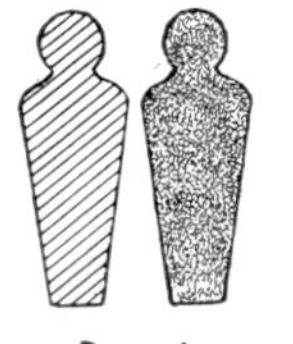

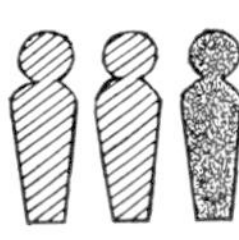

If two diabetics marry, all of their children will become diabetic eventually.

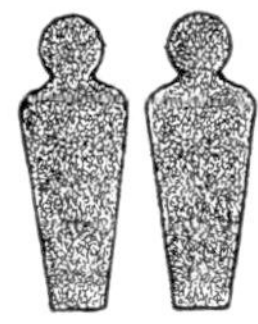

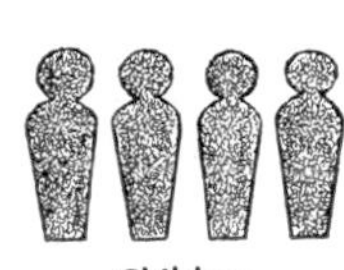

* Adapted from Forecast, American Diabetes Association, Inc., 1953.

FIGURE 3

build. (See Weight Charts, Appendix, pp. 189 to 191.)

DIABETES AND OBESITY

Statistics have shown that there is a definite relationship between the incidence of diabetes and obesity (Fig. 4). Although the exact reason for this association is not known, there is sufficient evidence to indicate that persons who are overweight are more vulnerable. One explanation that has been proposed is that with susceptible individuals an excess of food intake places demands upon the pancreas for an extra supply of insulin; this causes overactivity of the gland with eventual exhaustion resulting in diabetes.

There is general agreement that obesity is a health hazard, regardless of the presence of diabetes or other conditions. As overeating, in most instances, is the cause of obesity, care is necessary in the selection of food for the maintenance of desirable weight as well as for serving one's physical requirements.

AGE, SEX AND DIABETES

Diabetes can develop at any age. The highest incidence occurs from 40 to 60 years of age, while the percentage in infancy and childhood is comparatively small. Diabetes does occur in the 70's and the 80's, although the incidence is much lower than in the middle age group.

INCIDENCE OF OVERWEIGHT BEFORE ONSET OF DIABETES*

OUT OF EVERY **20** DIABETICS OVER 40 YEARS OF AGE,

17 WERE OVERWEIGHT BEFORE ONSET

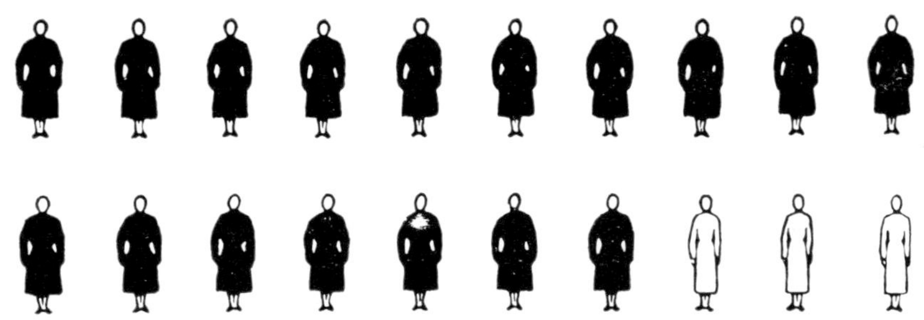

* Metropolitan Life Insurance Company.

FIGURE 4

TREATMENT FOR DIABETES*

It should always be a great comfort to patients to learn that there is definite treatment for diabetes which, when followed conscientiously, will help immeasurably in the achievement and the maintenance of controlled diabetes.

Factors in Treatment

No one plan of treatment can be prescribed for all patients, since requirements are determined on an individual basis. However, the treatment always includes a diet which contains adequate kinds and amounts of foods to supply food constituents for body needs. In many instances, in addition to the prescribed diet, insulin therapy, and/or the use of oral drugs, is needed for diabetic control. Together with these, treatment includes carefully regulated exercise, a regular routine in daily living, as well as special attention to personal hygiene.

* The patient and his family can obtain helpful information and learn of new knowledge about diabetes and its treatment by reading the American Diabetes Association publication FORECAST and also by joining the local Affiliate Diabetes Association.

Controlled Diabetes

The following standards have been established to describe controlled diabetes. These criteria should serve as a goal to be achieved whenever possible.

Weight: Maintained at desirable or ideal level (pp. 189 to 191).

Signs and Symptoms of Diabetes: Absent (p. 4).

Blood-Sugar Levels: Within reasonably normal limits (p. 3).

Urine Sugar: Little to none (p. 3).

Acidosis: Absent (p. 3).

Insulin Reactions: Absent (p. 3).

The treatment for diabetes must be followed every day all the patient's life, and no detail must be overlooked. Thus cared for and controlled, diabetes should not interfere with a full and normal way of life.

2. NORMAL AND DIABETIC DIETS

THE TREATMENT for diabetes always includes a carefully regulated diet. *This diet is individualized, and that which is applicable to one person is not always recommended for another.* Such factors as physical activity, present weight in relationship to ideal weight, the usual amount of food eaten, the severity of the diabetes and many other considerations all lend themselves to determining the best dietary treatment. The diet prescription must be determined by the physician, but the responsibility for adhering to the diet rests with the patient.

All diabetic diets have this in common—they must supply the proper kinds and amounts of the food nutrients to fulfill body needs and maintain an ideal weight. For this reason a knowledge of the normal diet is important. A discussion of essential dietary information follows. This discussion furnishes one with the fundamentals for understanding the diabetic diet and the information conducive to making that diet as flexible as possible within the dietary prescription.

THE NORMAL DIET

Everyone requires an adequate diet to maintain good health. An adequate diet, often called a protective diet, must contain proper amounts of certain food substances (p. 17). These substances, or nutrients, are carbohydrate, protein, fat, minerals (of which calcium and iron are especially important) and vitamins, particularly vitamin A, thiamine, riboflavin, niacin, ascorbic acid and vitamin D. The amounts of these food nutrients, together with the number of calories in the diet, are dependent upon the sex, the age, the height, the body build and the activity of the individual.

CARBOHYDRATE

STARCHES—SUGARS

For energy to work and play

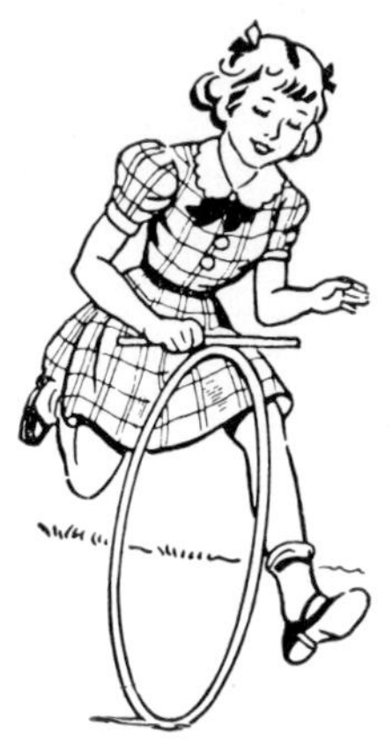

PROTEIN

For growth, muscle and repair

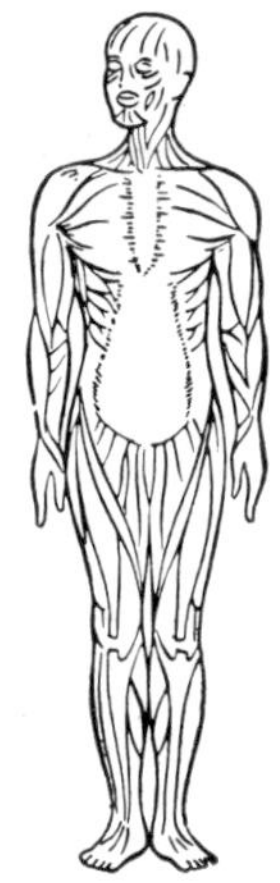

FAT

For energy to work and play

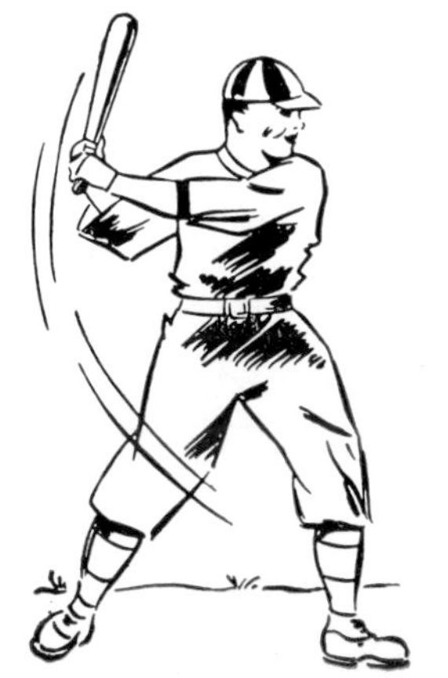

THE FOOD NUTRIENTS, FOODS THAT

Carbohydrate is the food nutrient that often is called a fuel food, for, when burned in the body, it provides the energy to work and to play. When taken in excess of energy needs, carbohydrate can be converted into fat which is then deposited in the body.

Carbohydrate is found in milk, bread, cereals, potato, rice, macaroni, dried peas and beans, other vegetables, fruit and fruit juices; in concentrated sweets* such as sugar, candy, jelly and honey; in desserts such as pie, cake and cookies; and in carbonated beverages.

Protein is the food nutrient that is necessary for growth, for building muscle and for repairing body tissue. Without protein there can be no growth and there can be no known life.

Protein is found in animal foods such as milk, cheese, eggs, meat and fish. It is also found in vegetable foods such as cereals, bread, dried peas and beans, potatoes and nuts.

Fat, also a fuel food, is again a food nutrient that provides the body with energy for its activity. When not used for that purpose, it is deposited in the body as fat.

Fat is found in dairy products, such as milk, cream, cheese and butter, in eggs, as well as in the fat of meat and fish, in nuts and in oils.

* Not used in the diabetic diet.

FIGURE 5

THEIR PURPOSE AND THE SUPPLY THEM

Calcium is the food nutrient that helps to build strong bones and teeth. It is the greatest part of the bone structure in the body and is also essential to the needs of the heart, the nerves and the muscles.

Calcium is found most abundantly in milk, cheese and other milk products; also in whole-grain bread and cereals; in vegetables, especially the dark green leafy ones; and in fruit, particularly oranges and the dried fruits.

CALCIUM
For bones and teeth

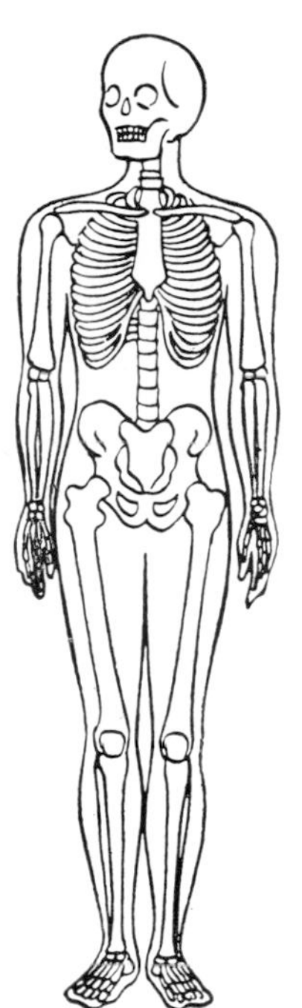

Iron is a food nutrient necessary for healthy blood. Iron is one of the factors responsible for the color and the condition of the blood. The blood carries food substances to every part of the body for the particular need of each part.

Iron is found in eggs, liver, lean meat, whole-grain and enriched bread and cereal; vegetables, especially dried or dark green leafy vegetables; dried fruits and molasses.

IRON
For blood

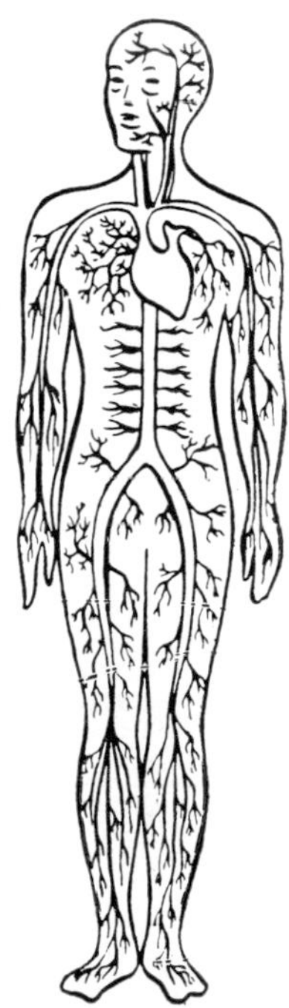

FIGURE 6

VITAMINS

FOR GROWTH, HEALTH AND VIGOR

Vitamin A is essential for the growth and the health of people of all ages. It is especially important in preventing night blindness and in helping the body to resist infection in the respiratory and the gastro-intestinal tracts. *The principal food sources of vitamin A are as follows:*

Dairy products (except nonfat milk)
Eggs
Liver
Fish-liver oils

Yellow vegetables:
- carrots
- sweet potato
- pumpkin
- winter squash

Green vegetables:
- kale
- spinach
- beet greens
- escarole
- endive
- broccoli

Fruits:
- cantaloupe
- apricots
- nectarines
- prunes
- peaches

Thiamine (vitamin B_1) helps to maintain and to stimulate the appetite, aids regular bowel movement, is essential in keeping the nerves and the muscles healthy and is necessary in the burning of carbohydrate. *The principal food sources of thiamine are as follows:*

Liver
Pork
Whole-grain and enriched cereals
Whole-grain and enriched breads
Potatoes
Peas
Beans
Green leafy vegetables
Fruits:
- oranges
- prunes
- bananas

Nuts

Riboflavin (vitamin B_2) is involved in the burning of carbohydrate in the body. It is necessary for growth, for good eyesight and for healthy skin. *The principal food sources of riboflavin are as follows:*

Milk
Cheese
Eggs
Lean meat, especially liver
Green leafy vegetables
Prunes

Niacin plays an important role in keeping the nerves and the body tissues healthy. *The principal food sources of niacin are as follows:*

Meat, especially liver
Poultry, especially light meat
Fish
Whole-grain and enriched cereals
Whole-grain and enriched breads
Potatoes
Peanuts
Peanut butter

Ascorbic acid (vitamin C) is essential for the normal development and the nutrition of bones, teeth and gums. It also helps to build and to maintain the strength of the walls of the small blood vessels. *The principal food sources of ascorbic acid are as follows:*

Fruit and fruit juices, especially:
- strawberries
- oranges and orange juice
- lemons and lemon juice
- limes and lime juice
- grapefruit and grapefruit juice
- cantaloupe
- tangerines and tangerine juice

Vegetables, especially:
- green pepper
- raw cabbage
- tomatoes
- spinach

Vitamin D assists the body in making the best use of calcium and phosphorus in the formation of bones and teeth. It also promotes growth and aids in the prevention of rickets. *The principal food sources of vitamin D are as follows:*

Milk, when fortified with vitamin D
Egg yolk
Fish-liver oils
Butter
Oily fish
Liver

FOODS THAT ARE THE PRINCIPAL

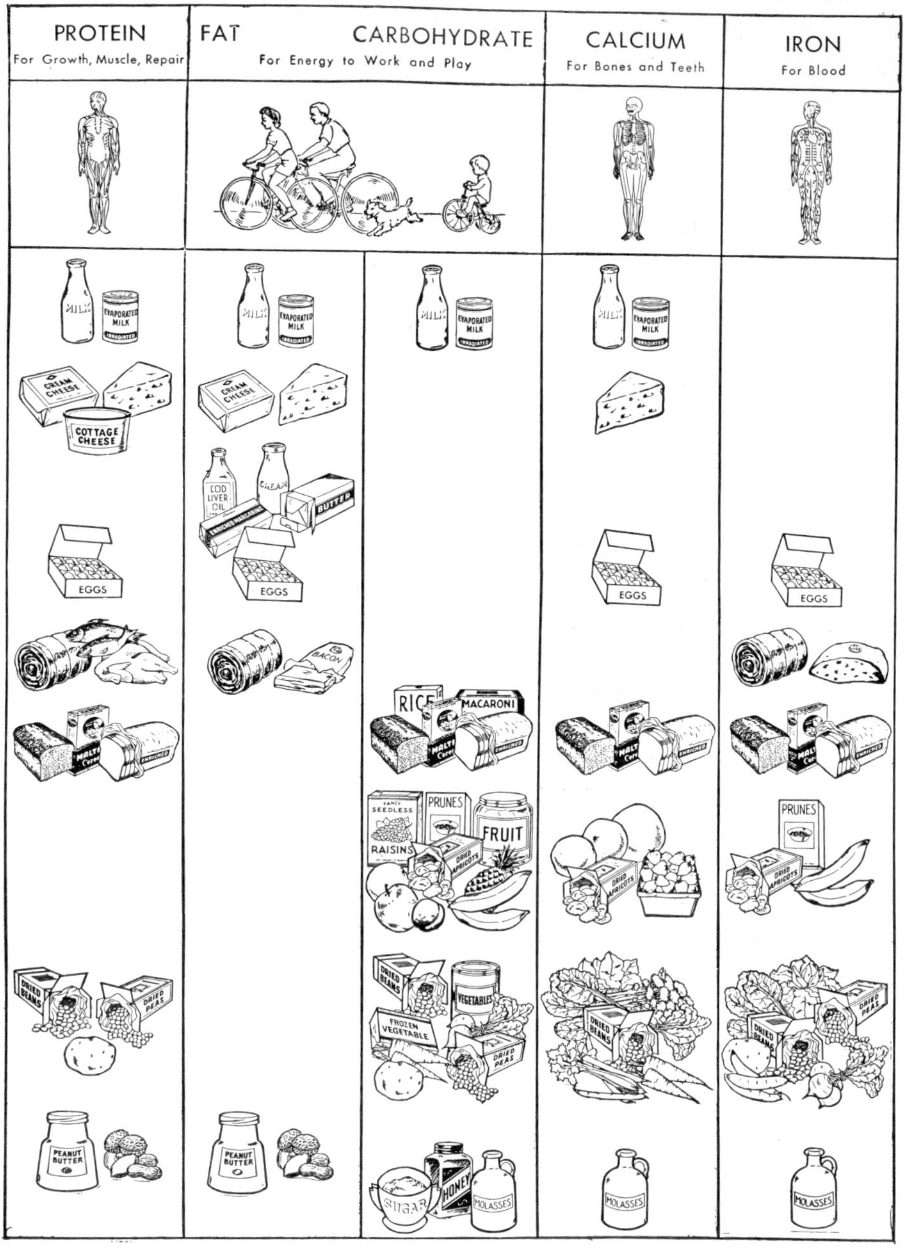

PROTEIN For Growth, Muscle, Repair	FAT For Energy to Work and Play	CARBOHYDRATE For Energy to Work and Play	CALCIUM For Bones and Teeth	IRON For Blood
MILK EVAPORATED MILK IRRADIATED	MILK EVAPORATED MILK IRRADIATED	MILK EVAPORATED MILK IRRADIATED	MILK EVAPORATED MILK IRRADIATED	
CREAM CHEESE COTTAGE CHEESE	CREAM CHEESE			
	COD LIVER OIL CREAM ENRICHED MARGARINE BUTTER			
EGGS	EGGS		EGGS	EGGS
	BACON			
MALT ENRICHED		RICE MACARONI MALT ENRICHED	MALT ENRICHED	MALT ENRICHED
		FANCY SEEDLESS RAISINS PRUNES FRUIT DRIED APRICOTS	DRIED APRICOTS	PRUNES DRIED APRICOTS
DRIED BEANS DRIED PEAS		DRIED BEANS VEGETABLES FROZEN VEGETABLE DRIED PEAS	DRIED BEANS	DRIED BEANS DRIED PEAS
PEANUT BUTTER	PEANUT BUTTER	SUGAR HONEY MOLASSES	MOLASSES	MOLASSES

FIGURE 7

SOURCES OF THE FOOD NUTRIENTS*

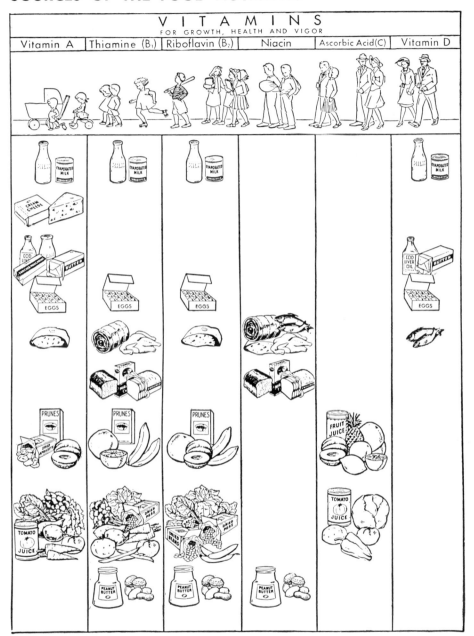

VITAMINS FOR GROWTH, HEALTH AND VIGOR					
Vitamin A	Thiamine (B_1)	Riboflavin (B_2)	Niacin	Ascorbic Acid (C)	Vitamin D

* Sugar, molasses, maple syrup, honey and other sweets are not used in the diabetic diet. (Prepared by the Frances Stern Nutrition Center in cooperation with the Maltex Co., Burlington, Vt.)

FOOD AND CALORIES

Through study and research, scientists have been able to determine the amounts of food nutrients which the body requires daily and also the number of calories needed for activity. Calorie is the term used to express the heat-producing value in food or, in other words, the amount of energy released when food is burned in the body.

Calories are furnished by only 3 of the food nutrients: carbohydrate, protein and fat. Minerals and vitamins do not supply calories. The body receives about 4 calories from every gram of carbohydrate; 4 calories per gram of protein; and about 9 calories per gram of fat.

Milk, which contains carbohydrate, protein and fat, is used as an example of calorie calculation. One glass of milk (8 ounces) contains 12 grams of carbohydrate, 8 grams of protein and 10 grams of fat. Since carbohydrate and protein supply 4 calories for every gram, then 48 calories are produced from the 12 grams of carbohydrate (12×4), and 32 calories from the 8 grams of protein (8×4). By using a similar method of calculation, 10×9 or 90 calories will be obtained from the fat. The number of calories from the carbohydrate, the protein and the fat in one glass of milk, $48 + 32 + 90$, when added will total 170 calories. The number of calories supplied from all foods can be determined in this manner.

Calories from certain carbohydrate foods such as sugar are called "empty calories," since they contain no other food nutrients. It is essential for the maintenance of health that the caloric requirement be supplied from the foods which contribute other food nutrients as well as calories.

The chart on pp. 14 and 15 shows, in summary, the various foods that are the principal sources of the food nutrients (Fig. 7). Note, for example, how many times milk, cheese, meat and other foods appear across the columns. These foods contain not just one but many nutrients. When a food supplies many nutrients, its contribution to the diet is valuable and therefore it is included in a protective diet (p. 17).

THE PROTECTIVE DIET
(The Normal Diet)

When certain groups of foods are included in the diet every day in certain amounts, the food nutrients necessary for the protection of health will be provided adequately. The protective diet, as this grouping of foods is called, is the basis and the guide for fulfilling the needs for all diets. Such a protective diet is shown below. (The recommended daily needs of the body in terms of specific nutrients are shown in Table 19, Appendix).

THE PROTECTIVE DIET—DAILY

Milk	1 pint for the adult 3 to 4 cups for the child
Egg	3 to 4 per week, adequate
Meat, fish or poultry	4 ounces ($\frac{1}{4}$ pound)
Fats	6 teaspoons of fat, including butter, margarine and other kinds of fats and oils
Fruits	At least 2 servings. A citrus fruit, cantaloupe or strawberries ensures adequate ascorbic acid.
Vegetables	At least 2 servings. A dark green vegetable ensures adequate vitamin A. Potato, if desired, in addition to other vegetables
Bread, Cereal, Crackers, Flour and Flour Products	6 or more servings, enriched or whole-grain
Sugar and Desserts	Amount dependent upon caloric needs

This is a general statement of the desirable amounts of food to provide the necessary nutrients and sufficient calories for the normal diet. However, it must be remembered that these amounts are listed for the normal diet, and that the diabetic patient usually uses less bread, cereal, crackers, flour and flour products, and potato. No sugar, candy or concentrated sweets should be used by the diabetic patient (p. 68).

THE DIABETIC DIET

The diet for the treatment of diabetes not only should supply adequate kinds and amounts of food to fulfill body needs but also must be a means of achieving or maintaining the ideal or desirable weight. Ideal weight is determined according to sex, age, height and body build. Standard charts with this information may be used as guides (Tables 15, 16, 17, Appendix, pp. 189-191).

The diabetic diet prescribed by the physician is based on the ideal weight in pounds, which is then converted into kilograms (Table 1), a measurement of the metric system. One kilogram equals 2.2 pounds.

The total food allowance is considered in relation to the patient's actual weight as compared with the ideal weight and also with the amount of the patient's physical activity. Sufficient food can then be allowed to supply the needed calories. The hard-working laborer probably will require more food to provide energy than the man in a sedentary occupation. Similarly, the woman in a sedentary occupation such as office work may need less food than one doing housework.

TABLE 1. CONVERSION OF POUNDS TO KILOGRAMS

2.2 Pounds = 1 Kilogram

POUNDS	KILOGRAMS	POUNDS	KILOGRAMS
22	10	120	55
25	11	125	57
30	13	130	59
35	16	135	61
40	18	140	64
45	20	145	66
50	22	150	68
55	25	155	70
60	27	160	73
65	29	165	75
70	32	170	77
75	34	175	79
85	39	180	82
95	43	185	84
105	48	190	86
110	50	195	89
115	52	200	91

THE FOOD NUTRIENTS IN THE DIABETIC DIET

The diabetic diet is much like that for the normal person, but there are a few changes which are most important. For the *adult* the diet contains normal amounts of the following food nutrients: protein, usually fat, minerals and vitamins. As a rule, carbohydrate is lower than normal (Table 2). For the *child* the diabetic diet contains normal amounts of all the food nutrients (Table 2). The total calories furnished by the diet is calculated to ensure sufficient caloric intake for physical activity. Sugar and concentrated sweets are excluded from the diabetic diet (p. 68).

Carbohydrate (Starches and Sugar)

Since all the carbohydrate in the diet is available as sugar in the body, the foods that supply carbohydrate need special attention. A definite amount of this food nutrient is determined by the physician, and any error in eating too much or too little can make the difference between success or failure in the prescribed treatment.

The carbohydrate for the *adult* must be lessened, usually to the extent of one half of the normal allowance (see Appendix, p. 194, Recommended Daily Needs). *Children,* with their needs for growth as well as activity, usually require amounts of carbohydrate within normal limits (see Appendix, p. 194, Recommended Daily Needs).

Protein

The protein allowances for both adults and children are usually the same as those recommended for the normal diet (see Appendix, p. 194, Recommended Daily Needs). The protein in the diet must be calculated, not only to ensure adequate amounts, but also because about 60% of the total amount of protein is converted into sugar in the body.

There are two kinds of protein: one is called "complete protein," and the other "incomplete protein." The former refers to such protein foods as milk, cheese, eggs, meat, fish and poultry. These are superior to incomplete protein foods which include breads, cereals, flour products and vegetables such as dried peas and beans and nuts. From one third to one half of the protein in the diet should be supplied from complete protein foods which are listed and illustrated on pages 30 to 33. The incomplete protein foods are included with the carbohydrate exchanges (pp. 42 to 49) or with the fat exchanges (pp. 34 to 37).

Fat

The fat prescription in the diabetic diet is usually within normal limits. Daily allowance of fat depends upon both the activity and the weight of the patient. Sometimes, as in the case of overweight people, the fat allowance may be lower than normal (see Appendix, p. 194, Recommended Daily Needs).

The function of fat, much like carbohydrate, is to furnish the body with energy. And, as fat contributes over twice as many calories per gram as carbohydrate and protein, the patient must not exceed the amount of fat prescribed.

Recent studies have indicated that the fat consumption per capita has increased significantly in this country since the first part of the 20th century. Some authorities believe that there may be a relationship between this increase in fat consumption and the high incidence of obesity, atherosclerosis and heart disease. It is also believed by some that the kinds of fat, as well as their proportions in the diet, may be important. Therefore, the practice of many physicians today is to modify the proportion of saturated and unsaturated fatty acids in the diet by using oil in place of butter, lean meats instead of meats having a high fat content, skim milk instead of whole milk, as well as a restriction of the amount of eggs and cheese allowed.

SUMMARY OF NORMAL AND DIABETIC DIETS

The following Table has been prepared to summarize the comparison of the food nutrients in the normal and diabetic diets:

TABLE 2. DAILY NEEDS FOR NORMAL AND DIABETIC DIETS

Food Nutrients	Normal Diet *Grams per Kilogram of Ideal Body Weight*		Diabetic Diet *Grams per Kilogram of Ideal Body Weight*	
	Adult	Child	Adult	Child
Carbohydrate	4 to 6	6 to 10	Usually ½ low Normal	Normal
Protein	1 to 1½	1 to 3	Normal	Normal
Fat	1 to 2	2 to 4	Usually low Normal	Normal
Minerals	*	*	Normal	Normal
Vitamins†	*	*	Normal	Normal

* See Recommended Daily Needs in the Appendix, page 195.

† Supplementary vitamins are indicated for diets containing less than 1,500 calories.

SAMPLE DIABETIC DIETS

Once the diet prescription has been determined by the physician, it is fulfilled, making certain to include the foods necessary for a protective diet (p. 17). The kinds and the amounts of foods selected for this purpose are shown in the following sample diabetic diets for the adult. The food exchanges (pp. 23 to 59) furnish the information needed for varying the diet.

TABLE 3. SAMPLE DAILY DIABETIC DIET FOR THE ADULT*

Milk, whole	2 glasses (1 pint) or exchanges
Cheese	1 ounce or exchange
Egg	1 or exchange
Meat, Fish or Poultry	4 ounces or exchanges
Butter	3 teaspoons or exchanges
Fruit	4 servings (include 1 good source ascorbic acid)
Vegetables, Group A	Unlimited amount
Group B	1 serving (include 1 dark green leafy vegetable)
Bread	5 slices or exchanges
Tea, Coffee, Clear Broth	As desired

* This diet contains approximately: 150 grams of carbohydrate
70 grams of protein
70 grams of fat
1,500 calories

TABLE 4. SAMPLE DAILY DIABETIC DIET FOR THE ADULT*

Milk, whole	1 glass (8 ounces) or exchange
Cheese	1 ounce or exchange
Egg	1 or exchange
Meat, Fish or Poultry	5 ounces or exchanges
Butter	4 teaspoons or exchanges
Fruit	5 servings (include 1 good source ascorbic acid)
Vegetables, Group A	Unlimited amount
Group B	1 serving (include 1 dark green leafy vegetable)
Potato	1 small or exchange
Cereal	1 serving or exchange
Bread	3 slices or exchanges
Tea, Coffee, Clear Broth	As desired

* This diet contains approximately: 150 grams of carbohydrate
70 grams of protein
70 grams of fat
1,500 calories

HOUSEHOLD WEIGHTS AND MEASURES

The amounts of foods in the daily diet are listed in terms of household weights and measures, such as teaspoons, tablespoons, cups, by size or number. These weights and measures are learned with surprising ease by constant use. The practice of using household measurements enables one to select sufficiently correct amounts of foods allowed in the diet with assurance and without the mandatory use of scales. Such time-saving methods help the patient to enjoy normal mealtimes with family and friends.

TABLE 5. HOUSEHOLD WEIGHTS AND MEASURES

1 gallon	=	4 quarts
1 quart	=	4 cups
1 cup	=	½ pint = 8 fluid ounces
2 cups	=	1 pint
2 pints	=	1 quart
3 teaspoons	=	1 tablespoon
2 tablespoons	=	1 fluid ounce
16 tablespoons	=	1 cup (standard measurement)
1 ounce	=	28 grams (approximately)
16 ounces	=	1 pound
A full spoonful approximates 1½ level spoonfuls		
A rounded spoonful approximates 2 level spoonfuls		
A heaping spoonful approximates 3 level spoonfuls		
1 saucedish approximates ½ cup		
1 full saucedish approximates ¾ cup		
1 heaping saucedish approximates from 1 to 1½ cups		
1 scant saucedish approximates ⅜ cup or ½ cup minus 2 tablespoons		

FOOD EXCHANGES

When a serving of one food is equal to a serving of another food in terms of its nutrient content, it may be exchanged for the other food and is known as a food exchange. Thus foods with equal amounts of carbohydrate *and/or* protein *and/or* fat may be exchanged for each other without changing the total amount of any of these three nutrients in the diet prescription. As an example, 1 small potato has approximately the same amount of carbohydrate and protein as 1 slice of bread. Therefore, the potato may be eaten in place of the bread and is considered a bread exchange.

Once the patient is familiar with the diet prescription in terms of the total food for the day, the use of food exchanges enables him to vary his diet. The exchanges, used daily, are readily learned, and a variety of available foods and combinations of foods may be chosen with confidence. With this information, the selection of food at home and away can be accomplished with ease within the limits of the prescribed diet.

Hundreds of meals need planning and preparation each year in nearly all households. The use of food exchanges enables the patient to partake of family meals without imposing excessive burdens on the housekeeper. Seasonal foods can be used and advantage can be taken of good buys or special food sales in the usual manner.

The various food exchanges are discussed on the following pages. Pictures as well as printed lists are presented to assist the patient in learning the many varieties and amounts of food that may be eaten. The index for the food exchanges is included for easy reference. Nutritive values for the exchanges and for additional foods can be found in the TABLE OF FOOD VALUES in the Appendix (pp. 196 to 208).

INDEX FOR FOOD EXCHANGE LISTS

MILK AND MILK PRODUCTS

The exchanges for milk will be given first consideration, since milk and milk products contain appreciable amounts of the three nutrients—carbohydrate, protein and fat. Milk is also an excellent source of calcium and phosphorus, as well as a good source of vitamin A, thiamine, riboflavin, niacin and vitamin D (when vitamin D has been added to the milk). Therefore, milk should be included in the diet, but only in the amount prescribed.

The milk exchanges have been divided into three groups: whole milk, nonfat milk and cheese. The whole milks contain 12 grams of carbohydrate, 8 grams of protein and 10 grams of fat per listed serving and are exchangeable one for the other. When nonfat milks are exchanged for whole milk, two fat exchanges, equal to 10 grams of fat, should be added to the diet because skimmed milk, buttermilk and other products in this second group contain little or no fat.

The cheeses, which contain little or no carbohydrate, may be exchanged for whole milk provided that additional carbohydrate be included in the diet. This exchange is most easily accomplished by adding an extra serving of fruit to the diet, since one serving of fruit or a fruit exchange contains about the same amount of carbohydrate as 8 ounces of whole milk.

When desired, one may make an exchange for milk by using the exchanges listed and pictured on the following pages.

Milk may be used as a beverage, in soups or chowders, with cereals or fruit or in cooking.

Milk Exchanges

Whole Milk

A milk exchange contains about 12 grams of carbohydrate, 8 grams of protein and 10 grams of fat, the amounts in 1 cup (8 ounces) of whole milk. Each of the following servings is equal to 1 cup of whole milk and may be exchanged, one for another.

Dried whole milk	4 tablespoons
Evaporated whole milk	½ cup
Goat's milk	1 cup
Whole milk, homogenized	1 cup
Yoghurt, plain	1 cup

Nonfat Milk

Each of the following servings of milk contains about 12 grams of carbohydrate and 8 grams of protein but little or no fat. Each serving may be used in exchange for 1 cup (8 ounces) of whole milk by adding 2 fat exchanges (10 grams of fat) to the diet.

Buttermilk	1 cup
Dried skimmed milk powder	3 tablespoons
Evaporated skimmed milk	½ cup
Skimmed milk	1 cup

Cheese*

Each of the following servings of cheese contains about 8 grams of protein and 10 grams of fat but little or no carbohydrate. Each serving may be used in exchange for 1 cup (8 ounces) of whole milk by adding 1 fruit exchange (10 grams of carbohydrate) to the diet.

American (process)	1 ounce
Camembert†	1 ounce
Cheddar	1 ounce
Cheddar cheese spread	3 tablespoons
Cottage†	2 rounded tablespoons (add 2 fat exchanges)
Edam	1 ounce
Limburger	1 ounce
Old English Spread	2 tablespoons
Parmesan, grated	4 tablespoons
Roquefort	1 ounce
Swiss	1 ounce

* Certain cheeses, such as cream cheese and cream cheese spread, have little protein or calcium but considerable fat. Therefore, they have not been included on the cheese exchange list but will be found on the list for fat exchanges. All cheeses contain less of the B complex vitamins. This factor should be given consideration when cheese is used consistently in exchange for milk.

† Cottage cheese and Camembert cheese also contain less calcium than milk and should not be used often as an exchange for milk.

MILK EXCHANGES

Whole Milk

Each of the following servings contains about 12 grams of carbohydrate, 8 grams of protein and 10 grams of fat and may be used in exchange for 1 cup (8 ounces) of whole milk.

Whole milk (homogenized)

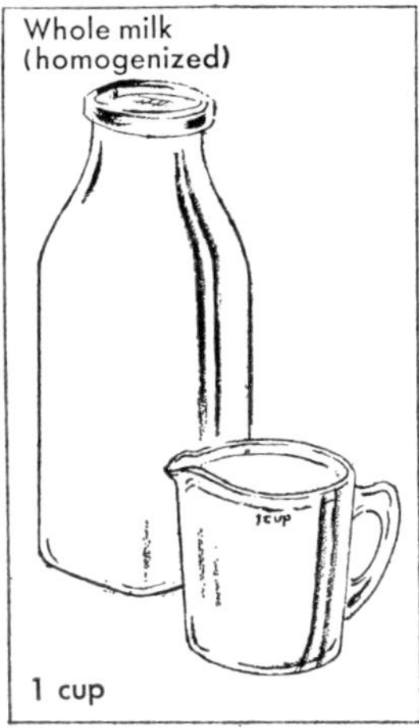

1 cup

Dried whole milk powder

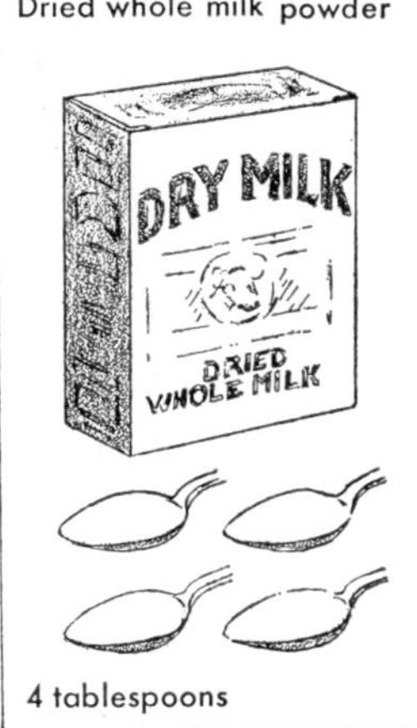

4 tablespoons

Evaporated whole milk

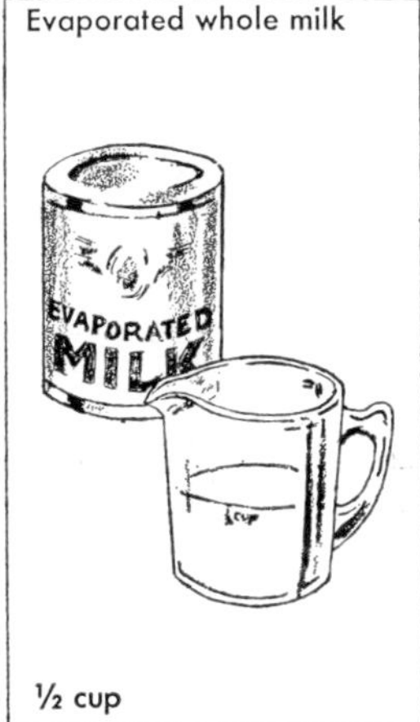

½ cup

Nonfat Milk

Each of the following servings contains about 12 grams of carbohydrate and 8 grams of protein but little or no fat. They may be used in exchange for 1 cup (8 ounces) of whole milk by adding 2 fat exchanges (10 grams of fat) to the diet.

Skimmed milk

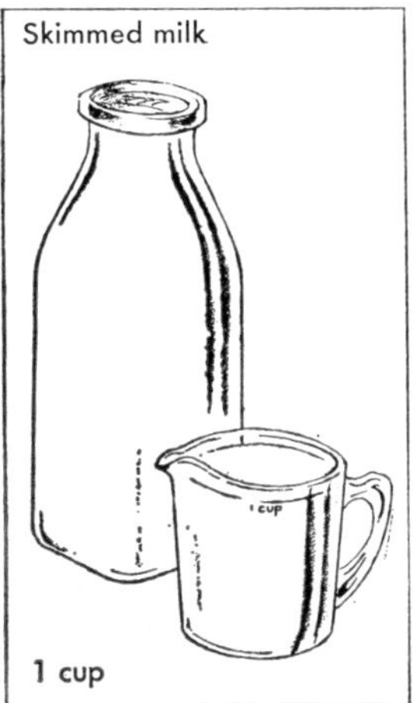

1 cup

Dried skimmed milk powder

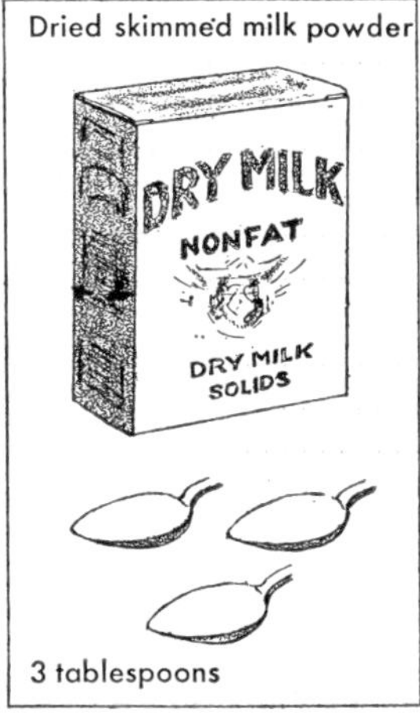

3 tablespoons

Evaporated skimmed milk

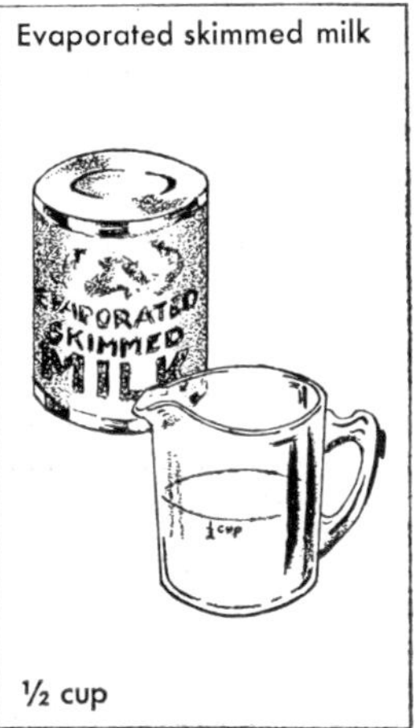

½ cup

Milk Exchanges

Cheese

Each of the following servings contains about 8 grams of protein and 10 grams of fat but little or no carbohydrate. They may be used in exchange for 1 cup of whole milk by adding one fruit exchange (10 grams of carbohydrate) to the diet.

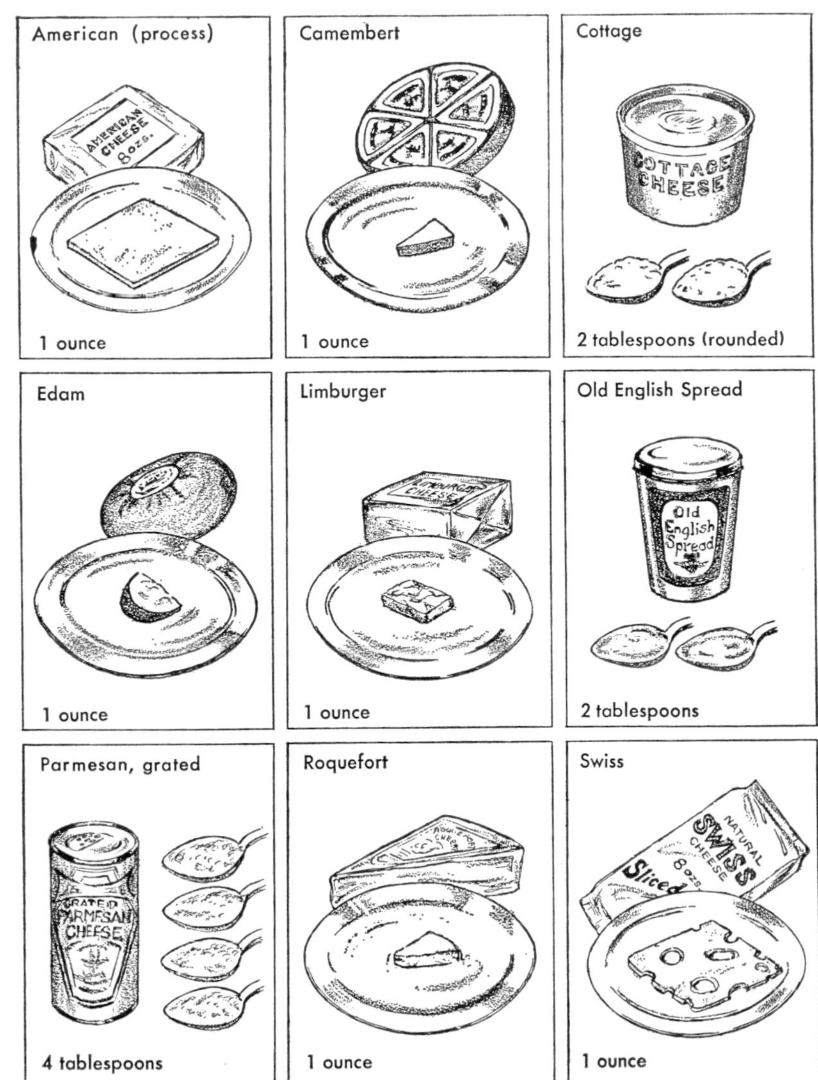
American (process)
AMERICAN CHEESE 8ozs.
1 ounce
Camembert
1 ounce
Cottage
COTTAGE CHEESE
2 tablespoons (rounded)
Edam
1 ounce
Limburger
1 ounce
Old English Spread
Old English Spread
2 tablespoons
Parmesan, grated
GRATED PARMESAN CHEESE
4 tablespoons
Roquefort
1 ounce
Swiss
NATURAL SWISS CHEESE 8 ozs.
Sliced
1 ounce

PROTEIN EXCHANGES

The protein contained in foods is important in the diabetic diet for two reasons. First, protein is necessary in all diets for the building and continued repair of body tissue. Second, it will be remembered that 60% of the protein in the diet can be converted into sugar by the body. Therefore, the same careful attention should be given to the amounts of protein foods in the diet as is given to the carbohydrate foods which are perhaps the more obvious sources of sugar.

The quality of protein is judged by the amino acids which it contains. Amino acids may be likened to building blocks, and when a protein food is "built" with all the amino acids essential to sustain life, it is called a *complete protein*. Complete protein foods come from animal sources and include milk, cheese, eggs, meat, fish and poultry. These foods contain little or no carbohydrate but do supply fat. From one third to one half of the protein allowance in the diabetic diet should be calculated to come from these complete protein food sources.

Incomplete protein is the term used to describe protein which is not "built," or made up, of all the essential amino acids, one or more of which may be missing. Thus an incomplete protein food, by itself, is not capable of sustaining life. Sources of incomplete protein are of plant origin and include foods such as bread, cereal, flour and flour products, nuts, potatoes and other vegetables. The carbohydrate content of most of these foods is high, and some of them such as nuts and peanut butter have a high fat content. When complete and incomplete protein foods are combined in the diet, as when one uses milk on his cereal, incomplete protein is supplemented by the complete form and together they enrich the diet.

However, complete and incomplete protein foods are generally not exchanged for one another, because of the differences in their carbohydrate content. For example, 1 egg contains 7 grams of complete protein and 5 grams of fat and may be exchanged for 1 ounce of meat, which also contains 7 grams of complete protein and 5 grams of fat. On the other hand, 1 egg may not be exchanged for a half cup serving of baked beans, which, although it contains 7 grams of protein (incomplete), contains large amounts of carbohydrate, like bread. Therefore, baked beans as well as most other incomplete protein foods with large amounts of carbohydrate have been included as carbohydrate exchanges and will be found on the bread exchange lists (pp. 46 to 49).

The protein exchange list that follows gives the kinds and amounts of complete protein foods that may be exchanged for 1 egg or 1 ounce of cooked meat. Although the fat content of most of the foods in the amounts given is about 5 grams, there are some, such as cottage cheese, the non-oily fishes and chicken, which contain almost no fat. Other exchanges, such as frankfurters and sausage contain more than 5 grams of fat. Unless exchanges for these foods are made frequently, the differences in fat content may be ignored.

In purchasing meat, fish or poultry it should be remembered that the amount of these foods allowed in the diet is in terms of *cooked* weight. Since meat, fish and poultry lose about 1/3 of their raw weight during cooking, the shopper needs to buy 1/3 more of these foods than is prescribed in the diet if the patient is to eat sufficient amounts. For instance, when the diet allows 6 ounces of cooked meat, 9 ounces of raw meat should be purchased (1/3 of 9 equals 3; 9 ounces minus the 3 ounces lost in cooking equals the prescribed 6 ounces of cooked meat).

Protein Exchanges

A protein exchange contains about 7 grams of protein and 5 grams of fat, the amounts in 1 egg or 1 ounce of cooked meat. Each of the following foods in the amount listed is equal to 1 egg or 1 ounce of cooked meat and may be exchanged one for another.

Cheese

American, cheddar or Swiss	1 ounce
Cottage	2 rounded tablespoons

Egg 1

Fish, cooked or canned

Anchovies	7 thin fillets
Cod	1 ounce
Flounder	1 ounce
Haddock	1 ounce
Halibut	1 ounce
Herring	1 ounce
Mackerel	1 ounce
Salmon	1 ounce or ¼ cup
Sardines	2 medium
Swordfish	1 ounce
Tuna	¼ cup, flaked

Fish, shellfish, cooked or canned

Clams	5 medium
Crab	¼ cup, flaked
Lobster meat	¼ cup
Oysters	4 medium
Scallops	1 large (12 pieces per pound)
Shrimp	5 medium

Meat and Poultry, cooked

Beef	1 ounce
Ham	1 ounce
Lamb	1 ounce
Liver and other organ meats	1 ounce
Pork	1 ounce
Poultry	1 ounce
Veal	1 ounce

Cold Cuts

Bologna	1 ounce or 1 slice
Cervelat	1 ounce or 1 slice
Liverwurst	1 ounce or 1 slice
Minced ham	1 ounce or 1 slice
Salami	1 ounce or 1 slice

Other Meats

Beef, dried, chipped	1 ounce (2 thin slices, 4″×5″)
Frankfurter	1 average
Sausage, pork	1 link (3″×½″)

Protein Exchanges

A protein exchange contains about 7 grams of protein and 5 grams of fat, the amounts in 1 egg or 1 ounce of cooked meat. Each of the following foods in the amount listed is equal to 1 egg or 1 ounce of cooked meat and may be exchanged one for another.

Cheese and Egg

American, cheddar or Swiss cheese

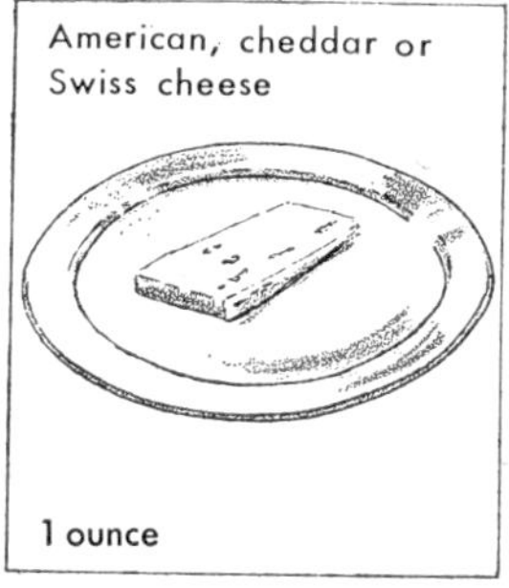

1 ounce

Cottage cheese

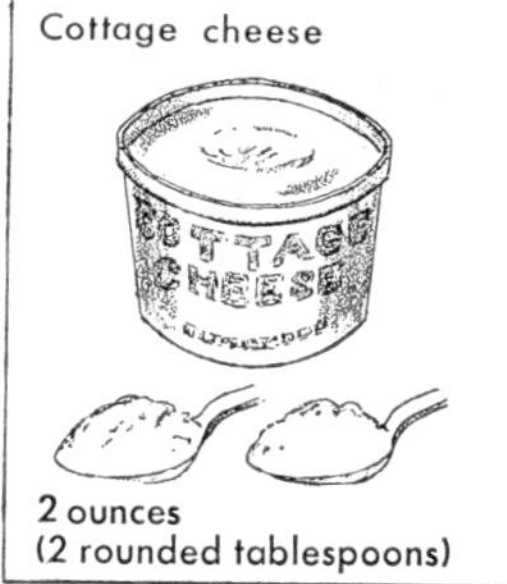

2 ounces
(2 rounded tablespoons)

Egg

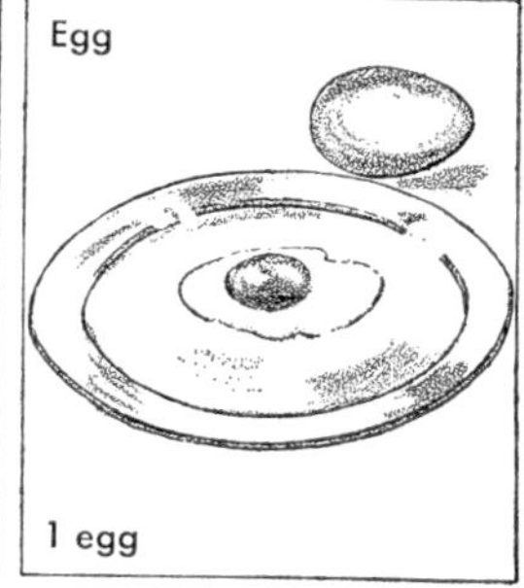

1 egg

Meat and Poultry

Bologna

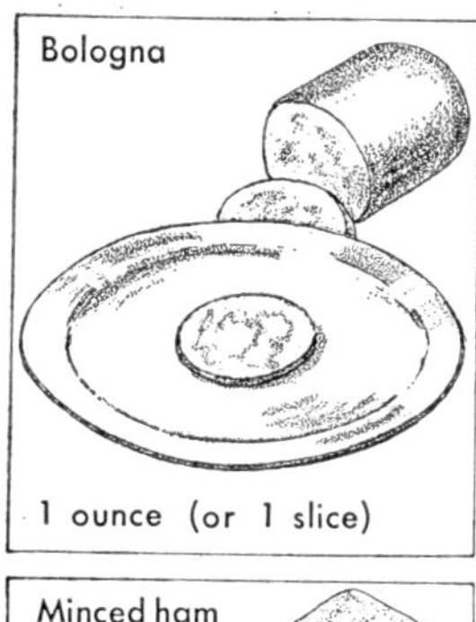

1 ounce (or 1 slice)

Frankfurter

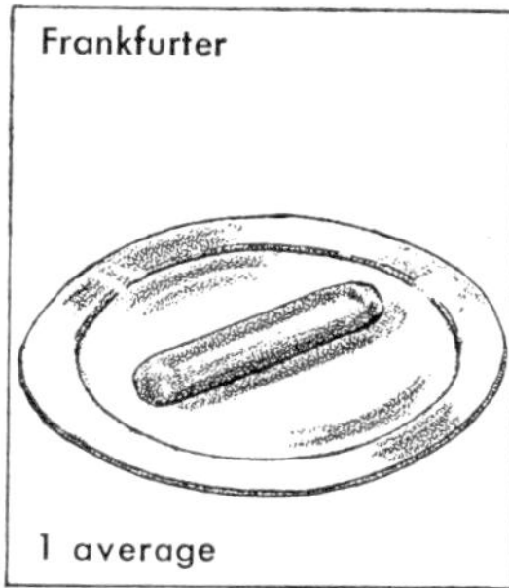

1 average

Meat

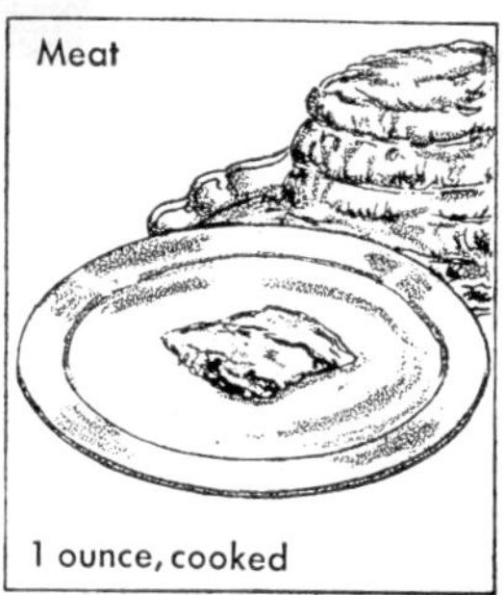

1 ounce, cooked

Minced ham

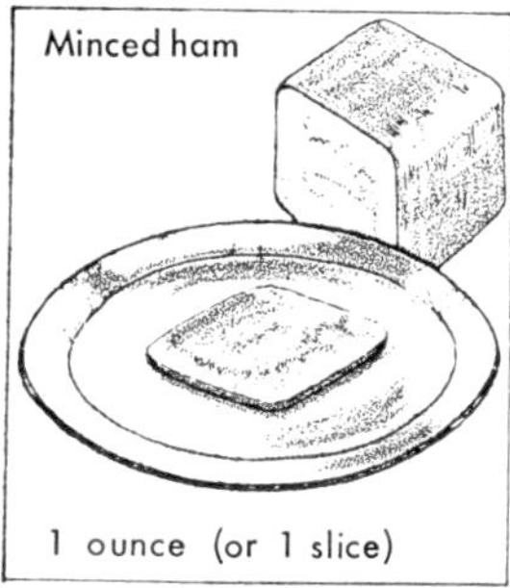

1 ounce (or 1 slice)

Poultry

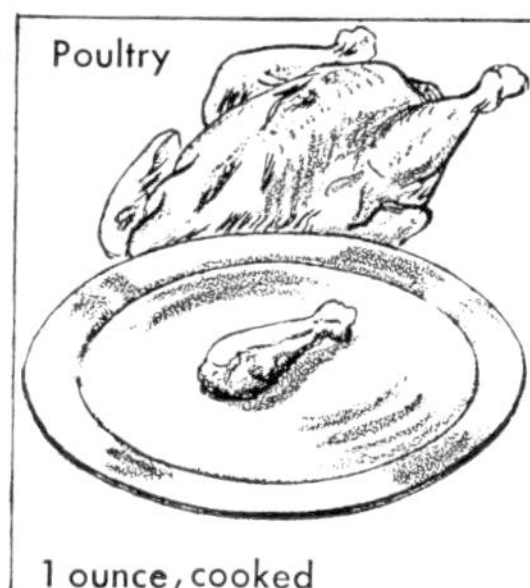

1 ounce, cooked

Sausage, pork

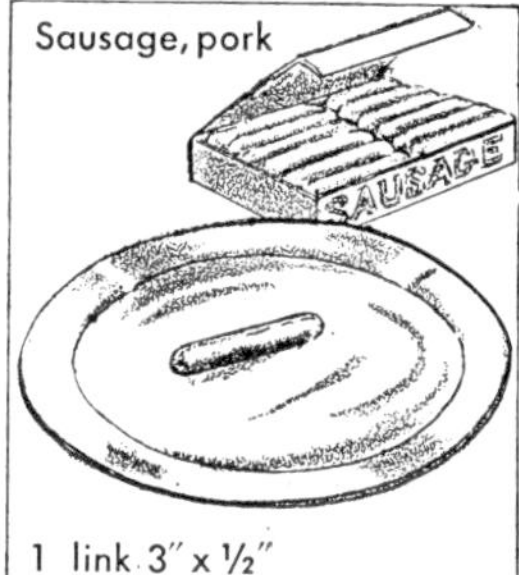

1 link 3″ x ½″

Protein Exchanges

A protein exchange contains about 7 grams of protein and 5 grams of fat, the amounts in 1 egg or 1 ounce of cooked meat. Each of the following foods in the amount listed is equal to 1 egg or 1 ounce of cooked meat and may be exchanged one for another.

Fish

Fish, cooked

(cod, flounder, haddock, halibut, herring, mackerel, salmon, sardine and swordfish.)

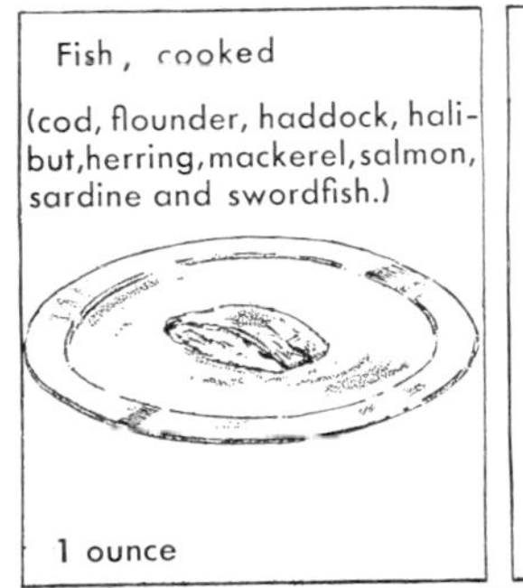

1 ounce

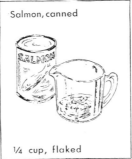

Salmon, canned

¼ cup, flaked

Tuna, canned

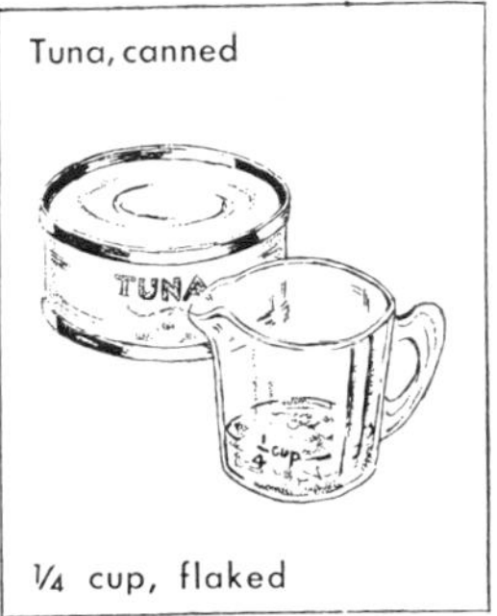

¼ cup, flaked

Shellfish

Clams

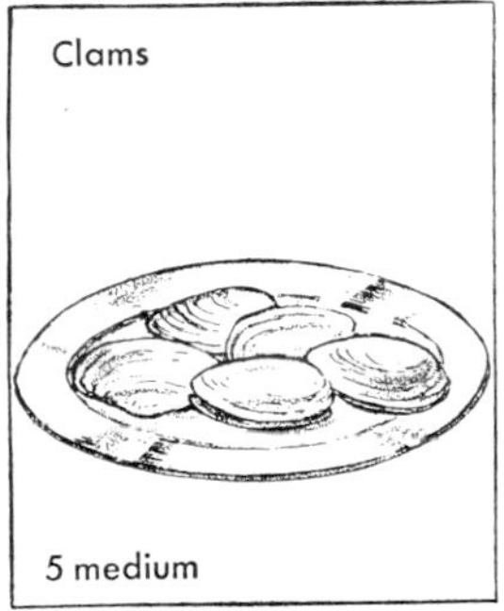

5 medium

Crab, cooked or canned

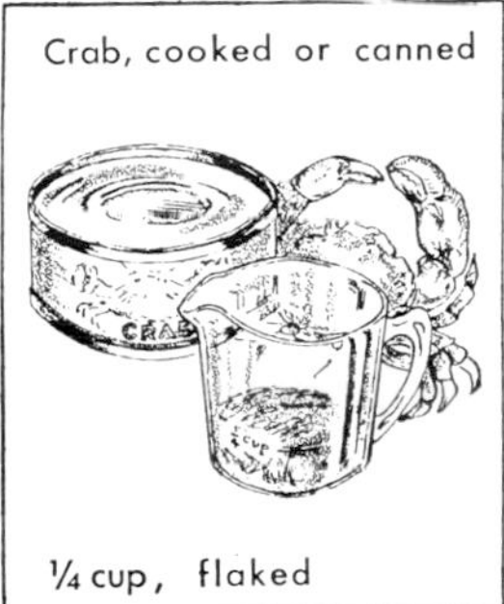

¼ cup, flaked

Lobster, cooked or canned

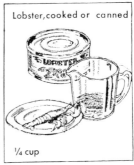

¼ cup

Oysters

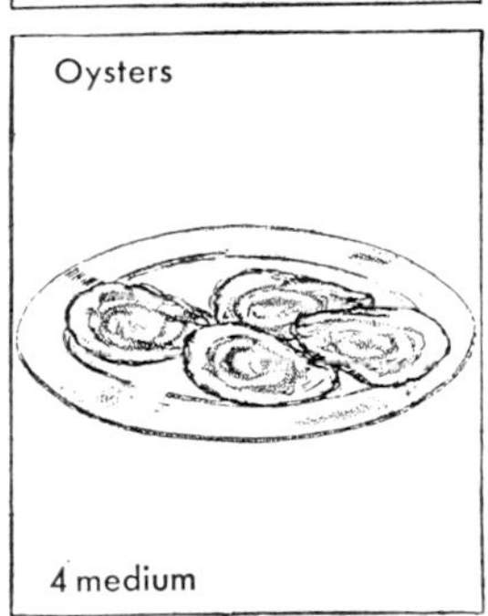

4 medium

Scallops

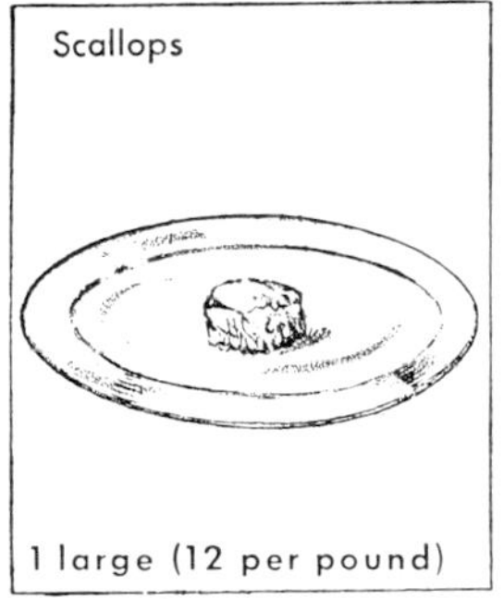

1 large (12 per pound)

Shrimp, cooked or canned

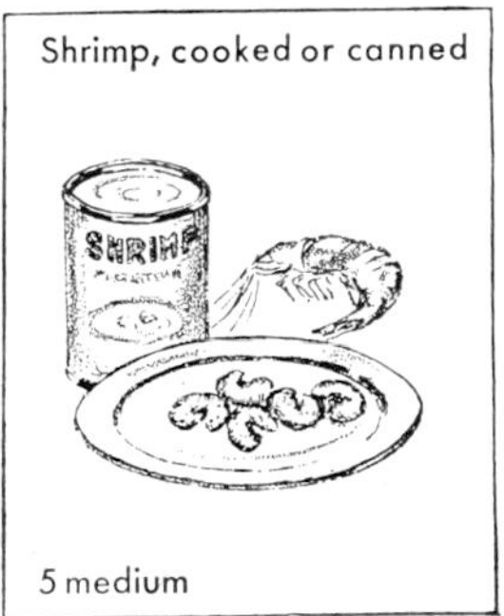

5 medium

FAT EXCHANGES

Certain foods contain almost all fat and little of the other food nutrients. These foods are commonly known as fat foods and are listed on the following pages as fat exchanges. There are some foods which, although they are considered primarily for their fat content, do contribute other nutrients to the diet. Butter, margarine and cream —the dairy fats—contain vitamins A and D; nuts and peanut butter contain appreciable amounts of protein as well as fat.

Nuts and peanut butter have been included in the fat exchange list because when they are used occasionally, or in small amounts equal to 1 fat exchange, they supply only small amounts of protein. However, when these foods are used frequently or in amounts greater than those equal to 1 fat exchange, their protein as well as fat content should be considered. For example, 2 teaspoons of peanut butter, the amount equal in fat to 1 teaspoon of butter or 1 fat exchange, also contains 3 grams of protein. This amount may be ignored when exchanged occasionally. However, when peanut butter is used often or in larger amounts, equal possibly to 3 fat exchanges, the total protein (9 grams) as well as the fat (15 grams) needs to be calculated.

The kinds and amounts of foods which contain approximately the same amount of fat found in 1 teaspoon of butter are presented in the following lists and illustrations.

Fat Exchanges

A fat exchange contains about 5 grams of fat, the amount in 1 teaspoon of butter. Each of the following foods in the amount listed is equal to 1 teaspoon of butter and may be exchanged one for another.

Dairy Fats

Butter or margarine	1 teaspoon
Cream, all purpose	1 tablespoon
Heavy	1 tablespoon
Light	2 tablespoons
Sour or cultured	2 tablespoons
Whipped, unsweetened	2 tablespoons
Cream cheese*	1 tablespoon
Cream cheese spread*	1 tablespoon

Fats and Oils

Bacon fat	1 teaspoon
Chicken fat	1 teaspoon
Cooking fat or shortening	1 teaspoon
Fat back	¾″ cube
Lard	1 teaspoon
Olive oil	1 teaspoon
Other salad or cooking oils	1 teaspoon
Salt pork	¾″ cube

Gravy and Sauces

Gravy, brown	2 tablespoons
Italian tomato sauce, plain	¼ cup
White sauce, medium	2 tablespoons

Miscellaneous Fat Foods

Avocado	⅛ small
Bacon, cooked, drained	1 full strip
Chocolate, unsweetened, melted	2 teaspoons
Olives, green or ripe	7 large
Peanut butter	2 teaspoons

Nuts

Almonds	8 nuts
Cashews	5 nuts
Peanuts	11 nuts
Pecans	6 halves
Walnuts	5 halves

Salad Dressings

French dressing	1 tablespoon
Mayonnaise	1 full teaspoon
Salad dressing (mayonnaise type)	1 tablespoon

* Certain cheeses, such as cream cheese and cream cheese spreads, have little protein and calcium but considerable fat. Therefore, they have been included here on the fat exchange list.

Fat Exchanges

A fat exchange contains about 5 grams of fat, the amount in 1 teaspoon of butter. Each of the following foods in the amount listed is equal to 1 teaspoon of butter and may be exchanged one for another.

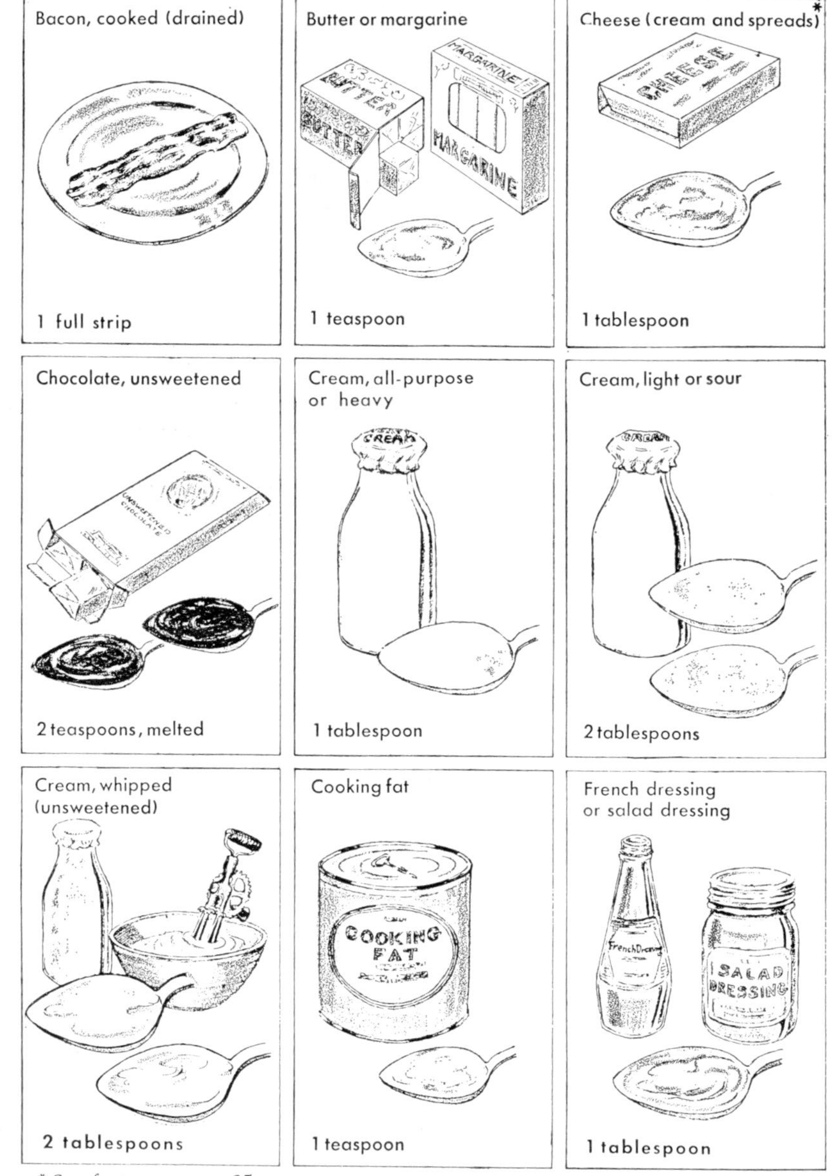
Bacon, cooked (drained)
1 full strip
Butter or margarine
BUTTER
MARGARINE
1 teaspoon
Cheese (cream and spreads)*
CHEESE
1 tablespoon
Chocolate, unsweetened
2 teaspoons, melted
Cream, all-purpose or heavy
CREAM
1 tablespoon
Cream, light or sour
2 tablespoons
Cream, whipped (unsweetened)
2 tablespoons
Cooking fat
COOKING FAT
1 teaspoon
French dressing or salad dressing
SALAD DRESSING
1 tablespoon

* See footnote on p. 35.

Fat Exchanges

A fat exchange contains about 5 grams of fat, the amount in 1 teaspoon of butter. Each of the following foods in the amount listed is equal to 1 teaspoon of butter and may be exchanged one for another.

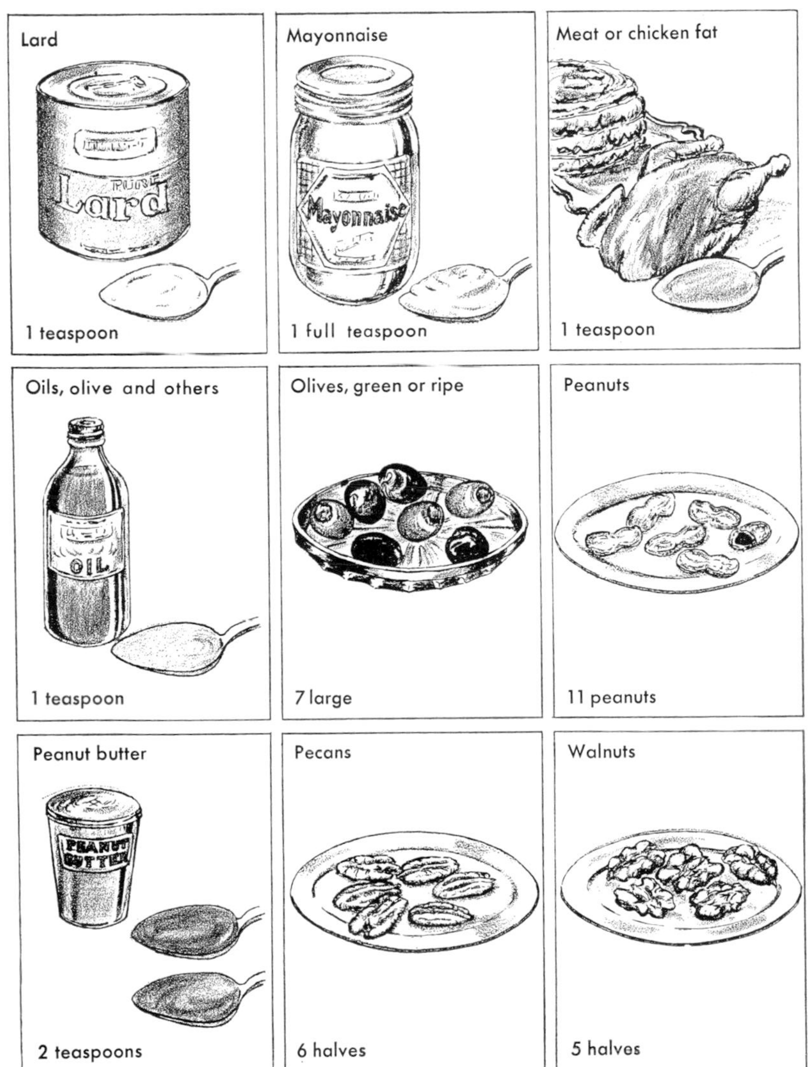
Lard
Lard
1 teaspoon
Mayonnaise
Mayonnaise
1 full teaspoon
Meat or chicken fat
1 teaspoon
Oils, olive and others
OIL
1 teaspoon
Olives, green or ripe
7 large
Peanuts
11 peanuts
Peanut butter
PEANUT BUTTER
2 teaspoons
Pecans
6 halves
Walnuts
5 halves

CARBOHYDRATE EXCHANGES—FRUIT

Fruits contain not only carbohydrate but other food nutrients, particularly the minerals, calcium and iron, and the vitamins ascorbic acid, vitamin A, thiamine and riboflavin. The amount of fruit allowed in the diabetic diet is determined by the carbohydrate content of the various fruits. A small orange measuring 2½ inches in diameter contains about 10 grams of carbohydrate or the amount in about 2 lumps of sugar. The following charts and illustrations list the various kinds and amounts of fruits that have the same quantity of carbohydrate as the orange (pp. 39 to 41).

These fruits may be exchanged, one for another, but it is important that one citrus fruit or other good source of ascorbic acid such as strawberries or cantaloupe be included in the diet every day to ensure an adequate intake of ascorbic acid.

Since all fruits contain carbohydrate or natural sugar, it should be remembered that the amount used is limited to that specified in the diet. Particular attention should be given to the size of the portions. For example, 1 small apple is listed as 1 serving of fruit. Therefore, when a medium apple is eaten, it must be considered as 2 servings of fruit or 2 fruit exchanges. The same principle applies to bananas and pears as well as to other fruits which easily can be taken in amounts that exceed the quantities prescribed.

Fruits may be eaten fresh, as purchased, or prepared in salads or fruit cup or as fruit juice; or they may be prepared with gelatin, baked or stewed without sugar. Cooked, canned or frozen fruits to which sugar or syrup has been added should not be used. Since most varieties of regular canned and frozen fruits do contain added sugar, labels on all containers should be carefully read for this information.

Carbohydrate Exchanges—Fruit

A fruit exchange contains about 10 grams of carbohydrate, the amount in 2 lumps of sugar. Each of the following foods in the amount listed is equal to 1 fruit exchange or 1 serving of fruit and may be exchanged one for another.

Apple	1 small
Apple	½ medium
Apple juice	⅓ cup
Applesauce, unsweetened	½ cup
Apricots, dried	4 small halves
Apricots, fresh	2 whole
Banana	½ small
Berries, average	½ cup
*Cantaloupe	½ of 4½″ diameter
*Cantaloupe	¼ of 6″ diameter
Cherries, sweet	15-18 small
Cherries, sweet	10 large
Cranberries, cooked, unsweetened	½ cup
Cranberry juice cocktail, unsweetened	2 cups (1 pint)
Dates, dried or fresh	2 medium
Figs, dried or fresh	1 medium
*Grapefruit	½ small
*Grapefruit juice, unsweetened	½ cup
Grapes, American varieties	15 (1 bunch)
Grapes, green seedless	40 (1 bunch)
Grape juice	¼ cup
Honeydew melon	¼ of 5″ diameter
*Lemon juice, unsweetened	¾ cup
*Lime juice, unsweetened	¾ cup
Nectarine	1 medium
*Orange	1 small
*Orange juice, unsweetened	½ cup
Peach	1 medium
Pear	½ medium
Pear	1 small
Pineapple, sliced	1 slice (3½″ × ¾″)
Pineapple, diced	½ cup
Pineapple juice, unsweetened	⅓ cup
Plums	2 medium
Prunes	2 medium
Prune juice, unsweetened	¼ cup
Raisins	1 full tablespoon
Rhubarb, cooked, unsweetened	1 cup
*Strawberries	13 large
*Tangerine	1 medium
*Tangerine juice, unsweetened	½ cup
Watermelon, cubed or balls	¾ cup
Watermelon	½ slice (10″×¾″)

* **Valuable as source of ascorbic acid (vitamin C).**

Carbohydrate Exchanges—Fruit

A fruit exchange contains about 10 grams of carbohydrate, the amount in 2 lumps of sugar. Each of the following foods in the amount listed is equal to 1 fruit exchange or 1 serving of fruit and may be exchanged one for another.

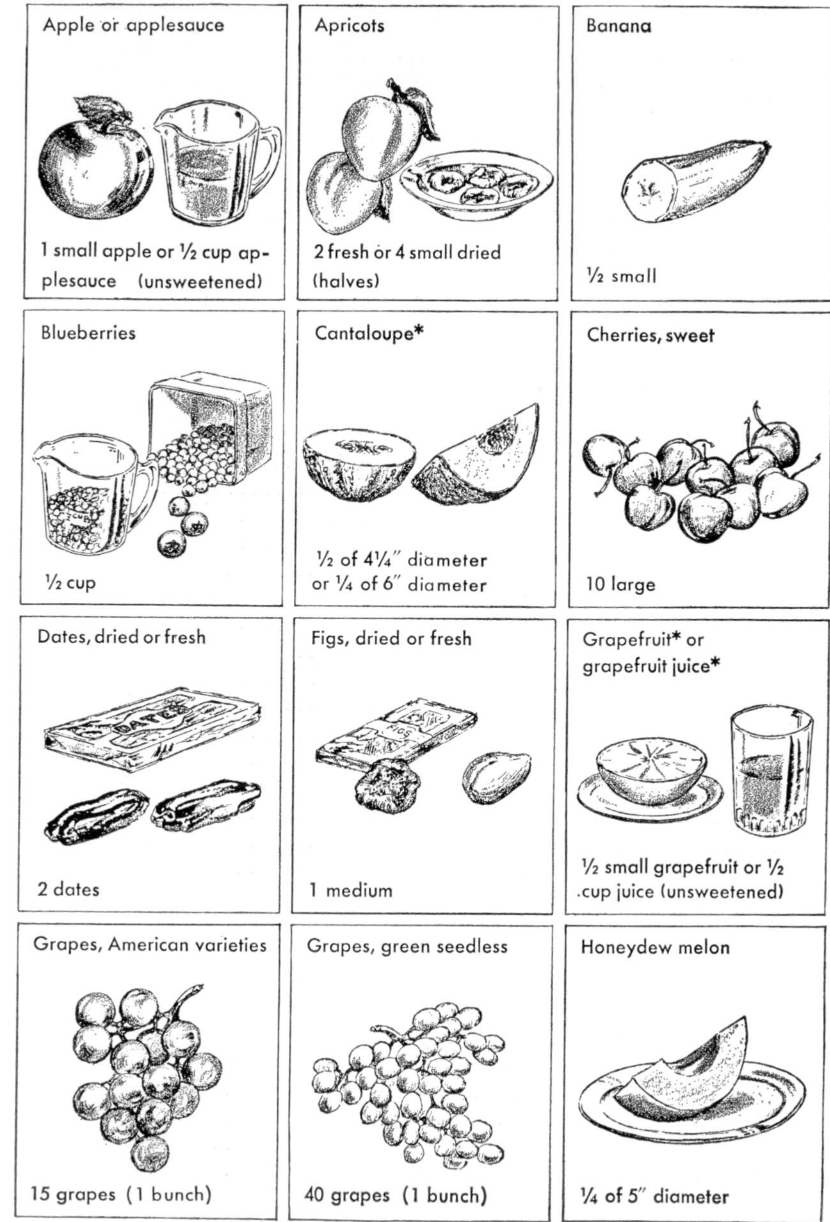

Apple or applesauce
1 small apple or ½ cup applesauce (unsweetened)
Apricots
2 fresh or 4 small dried (halves)
Banana
½ small
Blueberries
½ cup
Cantaloupe*
½ of 4¼″ diameter or ¼ of 6″ diameter
Cherries, sweet
10 large
Dates, dried or fresh
DATES
2 dates
Figs, dried or fresh
FIGS
1 medium
Grapefruit* or grapefruit juice*
½ small grapefruit or ½ cup juice (unsweetened)
Grapes, American varieties
15 grapes (1 bunch)
Grapes, green seedless
40 grapes (1 bunch)
Honeydew melon
¼ of 5″ diameter

* **Valuable as source of ascorbic acid (vitamin C).**

Carbohydrate Exchanges—Fruit

A fruit exchange contains about 10 grams of carbohydrate, the amount in 2 lumps of sugar. Each of the following foods in the amount listed is equal to 1 fruit exchange or 1 serving of fruit and may be exchanged one for another.

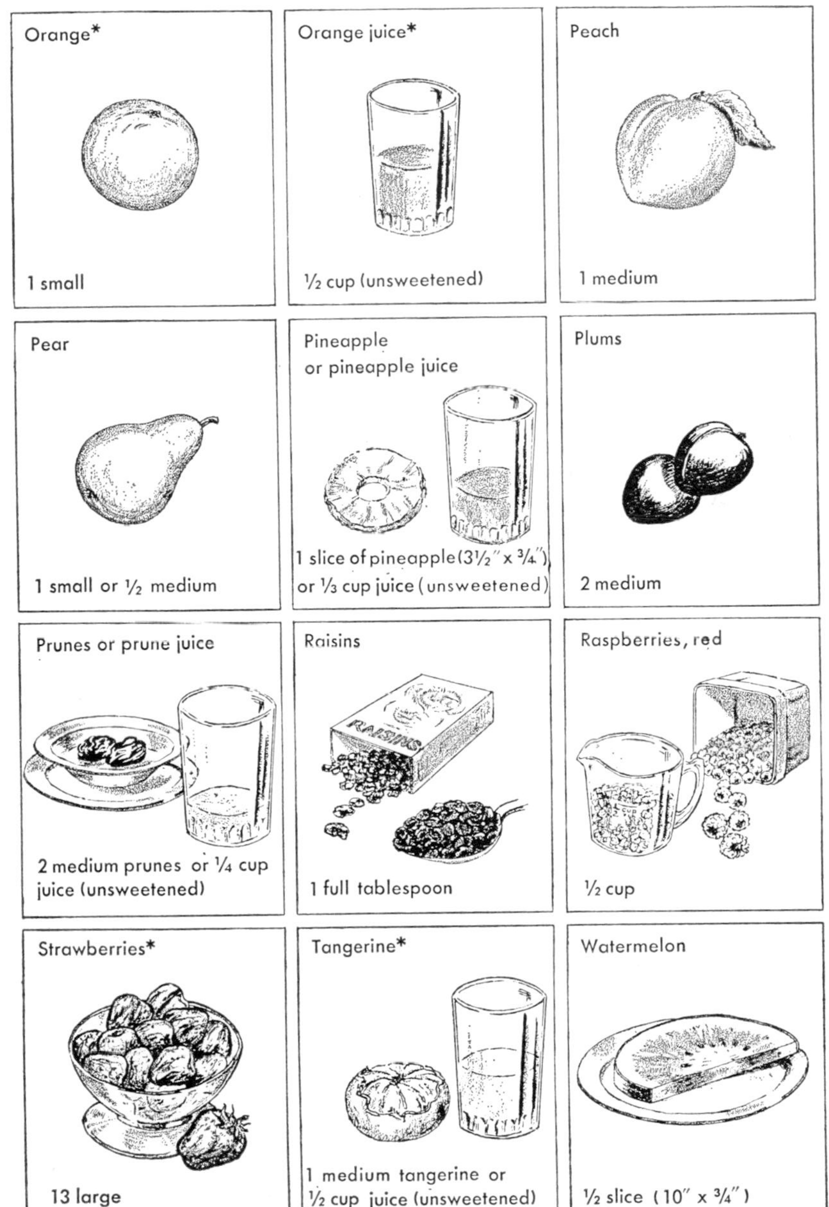
Orange*
1 small
Orange juice*
½ cup (unsweetened)
Peach
1 medium
Pear
1 small or ½ medium
Pineapple
or pineapple juice
1 slice of pineapple (3½" x ¾")
or ⅓ cup juice (unsweetened)
Plums
2 medium
Prunes or prune juice
2 medium prunes or ¼ cup
juice (unsweetened)
Raisins
RAISINS
1 full tablespoon
Raspberries, red
½ cup
Strawberries*
13 large
Tangerine*
1 medium tangerine or
½ cup juice (unsweetened)
Watermelon
½ slice (10" x ¾")

* Valuable as source of ascorbic acid (vitamin C).

CARBOHYDRATE EXCHANGES—VEGETABLES

Vegetables, like fruit, contain chiefly carbohydrate. They do supply a small amount of protein but no fat, usually, and are considered excellent sources of the minerals and vitamins. Vegetables are grouped according to the amount of carbohydrate that they contain, some having as little as 2 or 3 grams per serving and others having as much as 10 to 15 grams per serving. The vegetables that contain only small amounts of carbohydrate are listed as group A vegetables. They may be eaten freely by the patient to help satisfy the appetite, provided that excessive amounts are not taken. Eaten raw, an excessive intake of group A vegetables is not likely. However, when certain vegetables such as spinach are cooked, the volume is greatly reduced and the likelihood of eating excessive amounts is greater. The carbohydrate values of the group A vegetables can be found in the Table of Food Values in the Appendix (pp. 196 to 208).

The vegetables listed as group B vegetables contain larger amounts of carbohydrate and should be eaten only in the amounts prescribed. Vegetables that contain still higher percentages of carbohydrate than do the group B vegetables are included on the bread exchange list (p. 47).

Raw, cooked, canned or frozen vegetables may be used. They may be eaten plain or with butter, in soup, chowder or stew, in salads or sandwiches or in the preparation of "combination dishes" (p. 52).

Carbohydrate Exchanges—Vegetables

Group A

The following vegetables may be used in unlimited amounts:

Asparagus	Chicory	Pepper, green or red
Bamboo shoots	Cucumber	Pimento
Bean sprouts, mung	Eggplant	Radish
Beans, snap, green	Endive	Sauerkraut
Beans, snap, yellow or wax	Escarole	Spinach
Beet greens	Kale	Squash, summer
Broccoli	Lettuce	Tomato
Cabbage	Mushrooms	Tomato juice
Cauliflower	Mustard greens	Turnip greens
Celery	Okra	Watercress
Chard	Parsley	Zucchini

Group B

A Group B vegetable exchange contains about 10 grams of carbohydrate, the amount in 2 lumps of sugar, and 2 grams of protein. Each of the following foods in the amount listed is equal to 1 Group B vegetable exchange or 1 serving and may be exchanged one for another.

Beets, diced, cooked	¾ cup
Beets, whole, cooked	2 medium
Brussels sprouts	9 medium
Carrots, diced, cooked	1 cup
Carrots, cooked or raw	1 large
Collards, cooked	¾ cup
Dandelion greens, cooked	¾ cup
Onions	2 medium
Parsnip, cooked	½ cup
Parsnip, cooked or raw	½ medium
Peas, canned	½ cup, scant
Peas, fresh or frozen	½ cup
Pumpkin, cooked	½ cup
Rutabaga, diced, cooked	¾ cup
Squash, winter, cooked	½ cup
Turnip, diced, cooked	1 cup

Carbohydrate Exchanges—Vegetables

GROUP A

These vegetables may be eaten in unlimited amounts.

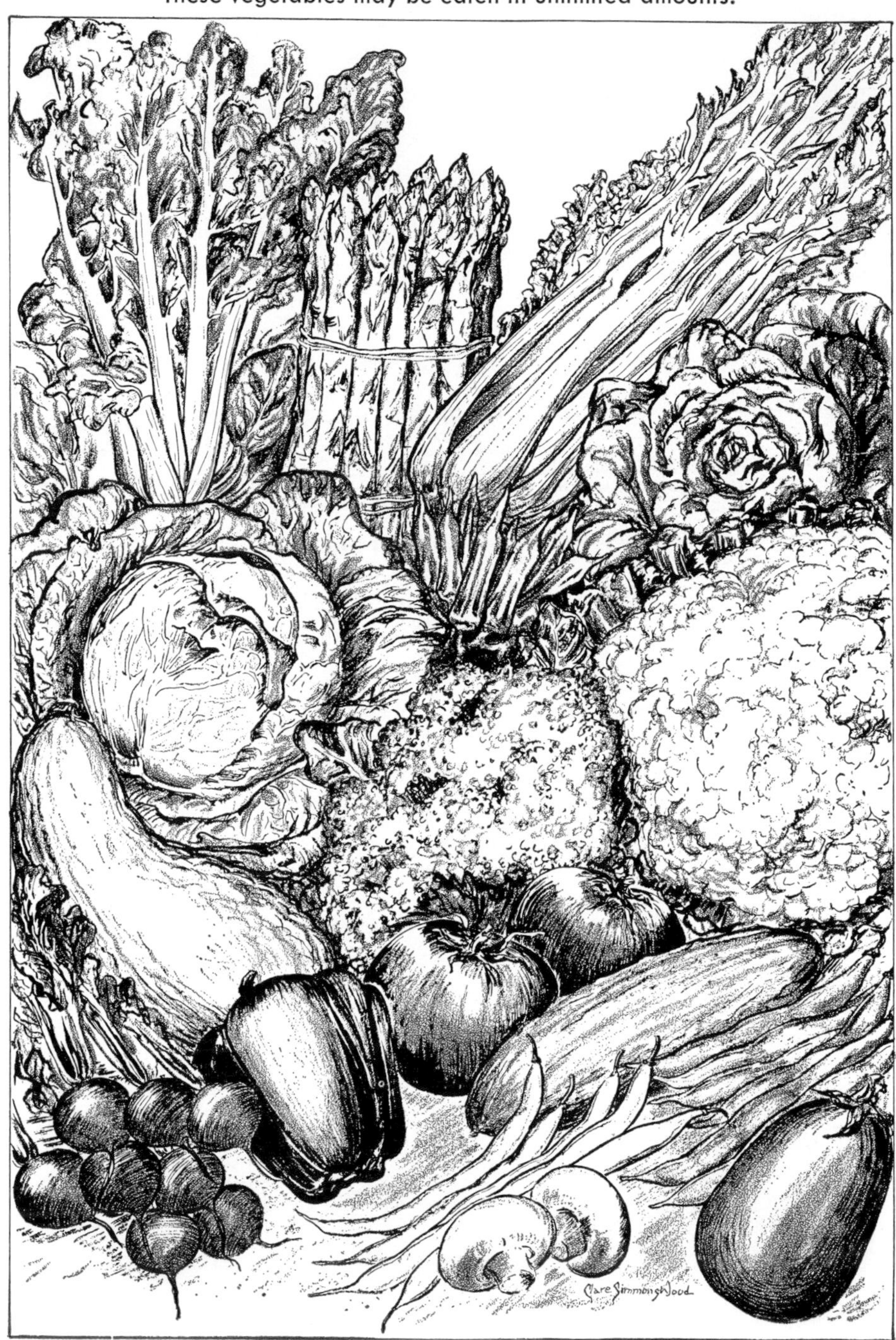

Carbohydrate Exchanges—Vegetables

GROUP B

A Group B vegetable exchange contains about 10 grams of carbohydrate, the amount in 2 lumps of sugar, and 2 grams of protein. Each of the following foods in the amount listed is equal to 1 Group B vegetable exchange or 1 serving and may be exchanged one for another.

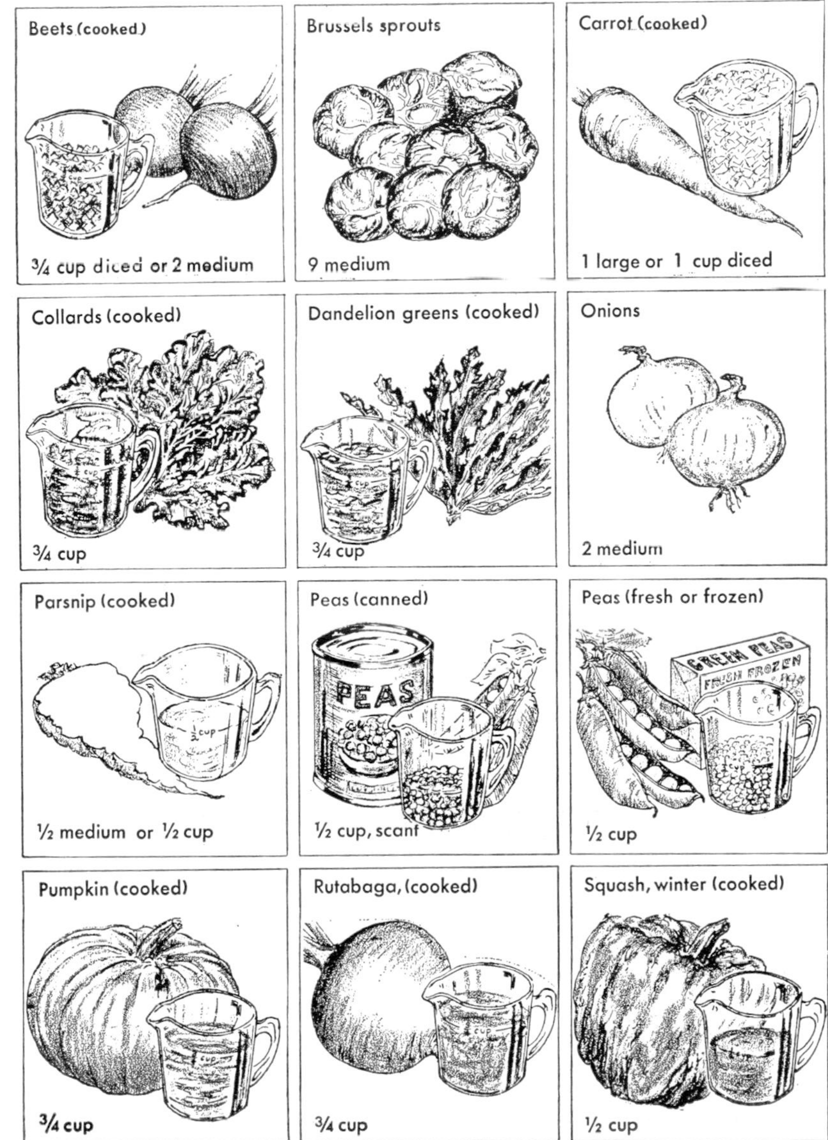

CARBOHYDRATE EXCHANGES—BREAD

Breads, Cereals, Crackers, Flour and Flour Products, Vegetables

Breads, cereals, crackers, macaroni, spaghetti and many similar products are made basically from the various grains and their flours, such as wheat, rye, oats and rice. Although these foods differ in ingredients, shape, texture and taste, they are considered as being exchangeable one for another, because of their similar carbohydrate content. Thus, one person may prefer white bread and another pumpernickel; one might eat rice, while another chooses macaroni; yet all would be eating food of essentially the same type and receiving approximately the same food value.

The following section of exchanges includes the many foods that comprise this group of grain products. They contain chiefly carbohydrate, small amounts of protein and little or no fat. The exchanges are based on the amount of carbohydrate contained in an average slice of American bread. This amount is approximately 15 grams, the amount in 3 lumps of sugar. The carbohydrate content of a slice of bread is the same whether fresh or toasted. Only the moisture content of bread is reduced in toasting.

There are many possibilities for varying the diet. Any one of the foods listed on the following pages may be exchanged for each slice of bread allowed in the diet. Vegetables which contain a high percentage of carbohydrate have been included with the bread exchanges rather than with the other vegetables whose carbohydrate content is lower. These are the group A and group B vegetables which have been discussed previously. A discussion of special breads such as "low calorie" or "high protein" will be found in the section on Food Fads (p. 70).

Carbohydrate Exchanges—Bread

A bread exchange contains about 15 grams of carbohydrate and 2 grams of protein, the amounts in 1 slice of bread. Each of the following foods in the amount listed is equal to 1 slice of bread and may be exchanged one for another.

Flour and Flour Products

Cornstarch . . . . 2 tablespoons
Flour, white . . . . 2 tablespoons
Macaroni, cooked . . . . ½ cup, scant
Noodles, egg, cooked . . . . ½ cup, scant
Spaghetti, cooked . . . . ½ cup, scant

Breads*

Bagel	½
Baking powder biscuit (2½" diameter)	½
Boston brown bread	1 slice (½" thick)
Bread crumbs, dry, grated	3 tablespoons
Bread sticks, thin (9" long)	4
Bulkie roll	½
Cornbread	1½" cube
French or Vienna bread	1 slice (1" thick)
Italian bread	1 slice (½" thick)
Melba toast	4 pieces
Muffin, plain (2¾" diameter)	½
Pumpernickel (4½" x 3½" x ⅜")	1 slice
Raisin bread	1 slice
Roll, frankfurter	½
hamburger	½
Parker House	1
Rye bread	1 slice
White bread	1 slice
Whole wheat bread	1 slice

Cereals and Cereal Products

Barley, dry	1½ tablespoons
Cereal, cooked	½ cup
Cheerios	¾ cup
Cornflakes	¾ cup
Corn, grits, cooked	½ cup
Corn, popped, plain	1½ cups
Grape-nuts	2 tablespoons
Grape nut flakes	½ cup
Muffets	1 biscuit
Puffed rice	1¼ cups
Puffed wheat	1½ cups
Rice, cooked	½ cup, scant
Rice, pre-cooked, dry	2 tablespoons
Rice flakes	½ cup
Rice Krispies	¾ cup
Shredded wheat	1 average
Tapioca, dry	2 tablespoons
Wheaties	¾ cup

Crackers

Animal crackers	8
Arrowroot	3
Butter thins	4
Cheese Tid-Bits	15
Chippers, potato crackers	4
Cracker meal	1½ tablespoons
Crax	4
Graham (2½" square)	3
Matzoth (square or round)	1 (6" diameter)
Matzoth meal	3 tablespoons
Melba toast	4 pieces
Milk (Royal Lunch)	1½
Oyster	20
Pilot (Crown)	1
Ritz, plain or cheese	4
Ry-Krisp (double square)	3
Saltines	4
Soda	3
Triangle thins	8
Triscuit	3
Uneeda Biscuit	3
Venus Wafers	4
Wheat thins	8
Zwieback	2

Vegetables

Beans, baked	2 full tablespoons
Beans, dried, cooked	¼ cup
Beans, Lima, cooked	½ cup, scant
Chickpeas, dry	1 full tablespoon
Corn, canned	½ cup
Corn, ear	1 small
Cowpeas, cooked	½ cup, scant
Peas, dried, cooked	½ cup, scant
Potato, sweet	½ small
Potato, white	1 small

---

* Breads of other nationalities may be used, provided that each slice is equal in size to 1 slice of American bread. The exchanges apply to toasted as well as fresh breads.

Carbohydrate Exchanges—Bread

A bread exchange contains about 15 grams of carbohydrate and 2 grams of protein, the amounts in 1 slice of bread. Each of the following foods in the amount listed is equal to 1 slice of bread and may be exchanged one for another.

Breads

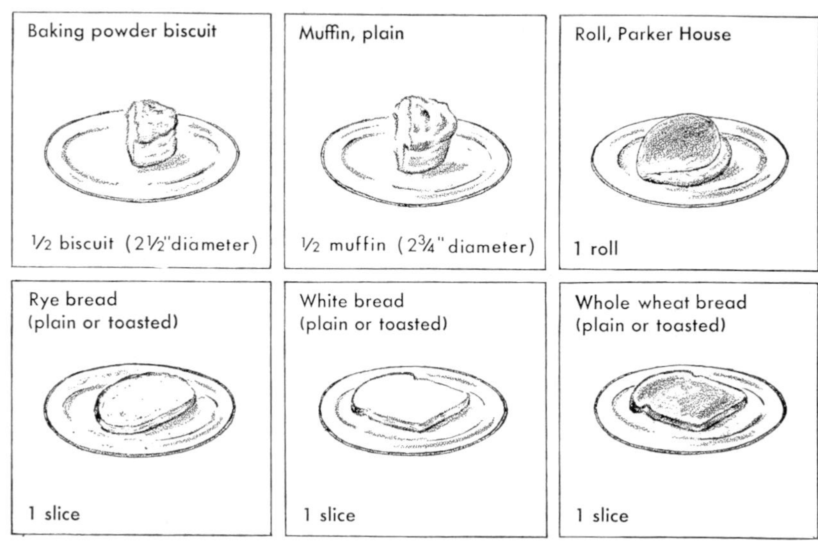

Cereal and Cereal Products

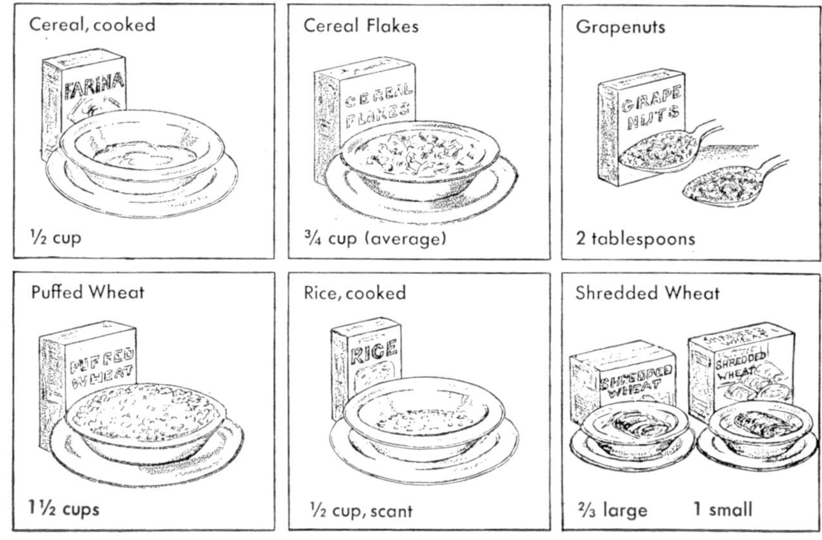

Cereal, cooked
FARINA
½ cup
Cereal Flakes
CEREAL FLAKES
¾ cup (average)
Grapenuts
GRAPE NUTS
2 tablespoons
Puffed Wheat
PUFFED WHEAT
1½ cups
Rice, cooked
RICE
½ cup, scant
Shredded Wheat
SHREDDED WHEAT
SHREDDED WHEAT
⅔ large
1 small

Carbohydrate Exchanges—Bread

A bread exchange contains about 15 grams of carbohydrate and 2 grams of protein, the amounts in 1 slice of bread. Each of the following foods in the amount listed is equal to 1 slice of bread and may be exchanged one for another.

Crackers

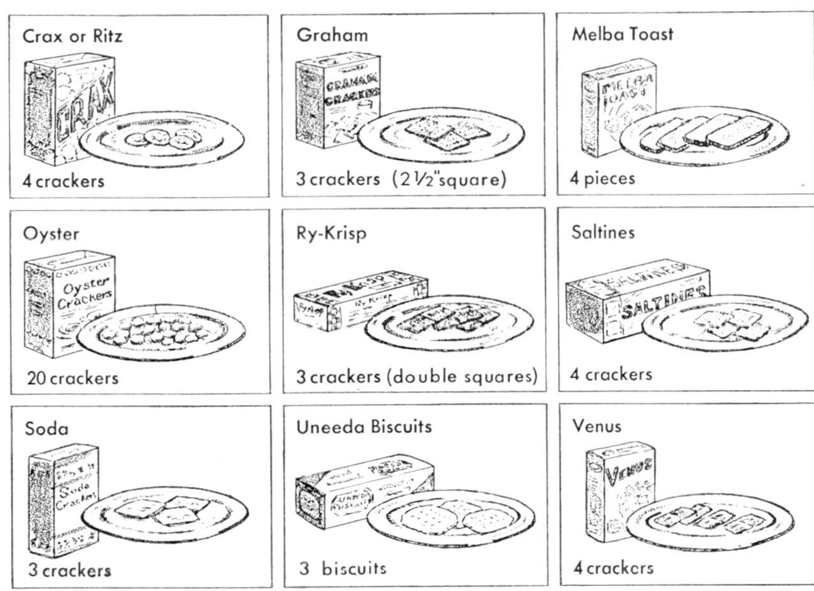

Flour and Flour Products

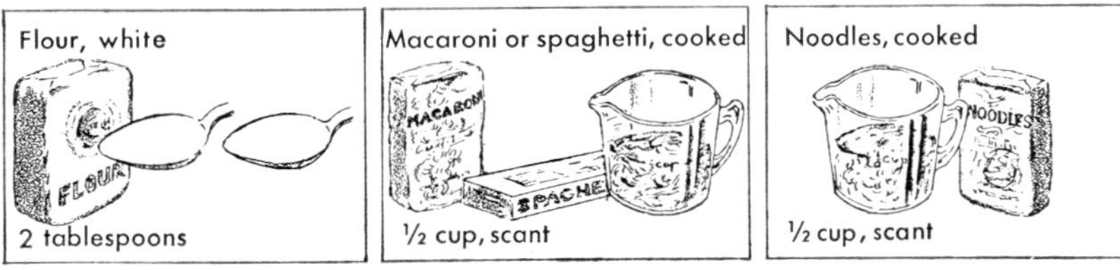
Flour, white
FLOUR
2 tablespoons
Macaroni or spaghetti, cooked
½ cup, scant
Noodles, cooked
½ cup, scant

Vegetables

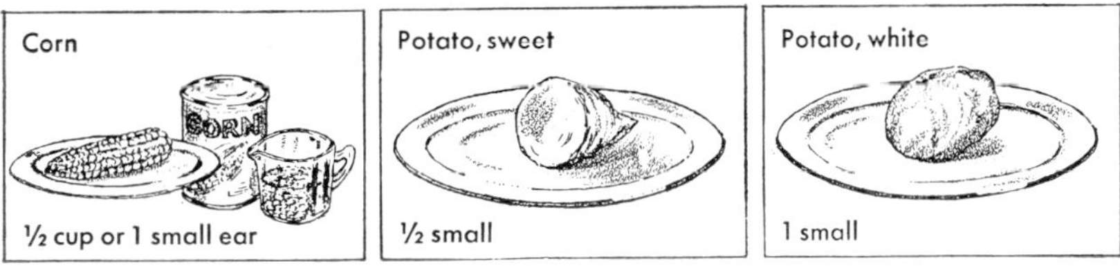
Corn
CORN
½ cup or 1 small ear
Potato, sweet
½ small
Potato, white
1 small

SOUP EXCHANGES

Canned, Frozen and Dehydrated

The diabetic patient may use soups, provided that the correct exchanges are made for their ingredients. Soups are wholesome, convenient and, for the most part, economical. For many, they serve as an important part of the meal. The use of a variety of soups helps in avoiding a stereotyped aspect to mealtimes as well as adding an extra course to the meal.

Canned, frozen and dehydrated soups contain varying amounts of carbohydrate, protein and fat. Therefore, the food exchanges will vary, depending on the amounts of these three nutrients in each variety of soup. For instance, the carbohydrate, protein and fat content of beef soup is similar to that of bread and meat and therefore, ½ can of condensed beef soup is exchangeable for 1 slice of bread and 1 ounce of meat (1 bread and 1 protein exchange).

The exchanges for condensed soups, both canned and frozen, are based on ½ can of condensed soup before water or milk has been added. When, in preparation, the soup is diluted with water, no food value is added; it remains the same. When milk is added, the food value is increased by the amount added which then must be considered as part of the milk allowance for the day.

The exchanges listed for the dehydrated soups represent the reconstituted amount or, in other words, the amount obtained after the soups are prepared with water according to the directions on the package.

Various garnishes may be used with soups to enhance their appeal and yet not increase their food value. For example, a few finely diced or shredded vegetables added to broth or consommé makes it more interesting to eat, or a slice of lemon, or lemon sprinkled with parsley and floated on the surface, is attractive and adds a distinctive flavor.

Soup Exchanges

The following soups may be used in unlimited amounts:

Bouillon; Consommé; Clear Broth

Other soups may be used in exchange for foods already allowed in the diet. The following list shows the exchanges which may be used for ½ can of condensed soup (before water or milk has been added).

Condensed Canned Soups	Food Exchanges
Beef	1 bread + 1 protein
Beef Noodle	1 bread
Black Bean	2 bread
Chicken Gumbo	1 bread
Chicken Noodle	1 bread
Chicken Rice	1 bread
Chicken Vegetable	1 bread + 1 fat
Clam Chowder, Manhattan style	1 bread + 1 fat
Cream of Asparagus	1 bread
Cream of Celery	1 bread + 1 fat
Cream of Chicken	1 bread + 1 fat
Cream of Mushroom	1 bread + 2 fat
Green Split Pea	2 bread + 1 fat
Minestrone	1 bread + 1 protein
Onion	1 bread
Scotch Broth	1 bread + 1 protein
Tomato	1 bread + 1 fat
Turkey Noodle	1 bread + 1 fat
Vegetable Beef	1 group B vegetable + 1 protein
Vegetarian Vegetable	1 bread

Condensed Frozen Soups	Food Exchanges
Clam Chowder, New England style	1 bread + 2 fat
Cream of Potato	1 bread + 1 fat
Cream of Shrimp	1 bread + 1 protein + 1 fat
Green Pea With Ham	2 bread + 1 fat
Oyster Stew	1 bread + 1 protein

The following list shows the exchanges which may be used for 1 cup of soup made from dehydrated mixes (after water has been added according to directions on the package).

Dehydrated Soup Mixes	Food Exchanges
Beef Noodle	1 bread
Chicken Noodle	1 bread
Chicken Rice	1 bread
Green Pea	2 bread
Onion	½ bread
Tomato Vegetable With Noodles	1 bread

EXCHANGES FOR COMBINATION DISHES

Many of the foods or their exchanges allowed in the diet may be combined, providing variety in the meals at home and also facilitating the selection of meals from restaurant menus.

When preparing combination dishes, the total food value of the ingredients, represented by the exchanges, must be estimated and appropriate allowances made for them. Macaroni and cheese is used as an example. Although this dish does not appear as such on the diet list, the proper exchanges can be made when the ingredients are known. Macaroni and cheese usually is prepared with macaroni, cheese, milk and possibly some fat and flour. The exchange can be accomplished in the following way. A scant ½ cup of cooked macaroni has about the same food value as a slice of bread. The cheese content represents one of the protein exchanges and the milk used may be deducted from the daily milk allotment. Since ½ cup of macaroni is rather a small serving, a whole cup may be used, representing 2 bread exchanges. This amount of macaroni would have about 1 ounce of cheese and 1 cup of milk in combination with it. Therefore, the total exchange needed for this dish is: 2 bread exchanges, 1 protein exchange and 1 cup of milk. With the omission of these items from the total daily food allowance, the correct exchange is completed.

Similarly, other combination dishes may be prepared and eaten by making the appropriate exchanges for their various food ingredients. Some of the more popular dishes are listed and illustrated on the pages that follow. It is hoped that the use of these will not only increase mealtime pleasure but also encourage the patient to add to the dietary list other dishes of his own creations and choice.

Exchanges for Combination Dishes*

Certain combination dishes may be included in the diet when they are used in exchange for the foods that are allowed. There are many combinations of foods which could be used, but space permits only the inclusion of some of the more popular ones. The following list shows how combination dishes can be exchanged.

Combination Dishes	Amount	Food Exchanges
Beef Stew	1 cup	2 protein 1 bread
Baked Beans and Frankfurters		
Frankfurters	2	2 protein
Baked Beans	4 full tablespoons	2 bread
Baked Macaroni and Cheese	1 cup	1 milk 1 protein 2 bread
Corned Beef Hash (Canned)	¾ cup	2 protein 1 bread 2 fat
Coleslaw	½ cup	1 vegetable (Group A) 1 fat
Italian Spaghetti	1 serving (1 cup spaghetti, 2 small meat balls, ½ cup sauce)	2½ bread 3 protein 2 fat
Chop Suey (Meat, Canned)	1 cup	1 bread 1 protein
Pancakes	2 pancakes (4″ diameter)	1 bread 1 fat
French-Fried Potatoes	5 pieces, 2″×½″×½″	1 bread 1 fat
Potato Chips	15 medium, 2″ diameter or 10 large, 3″ diameter	1 bread 2 fat
Poultry With Stuffing	4 ounces poultry ⅓ cup stuffing	4 protein 1 bread 1 fat
Chili Con Carne With Beans	1 cup	2 protein 2 bread

* Exchanges have been computed from figures in U. S. Handbook No. 8. Italian Spaghetti—computed from basic recipe.

Exchanges for Combination Dishes*

Each of the following combination dishes may be used, provided that the proper food exchanges are made.

Combination Dishes **Food Exchanges**

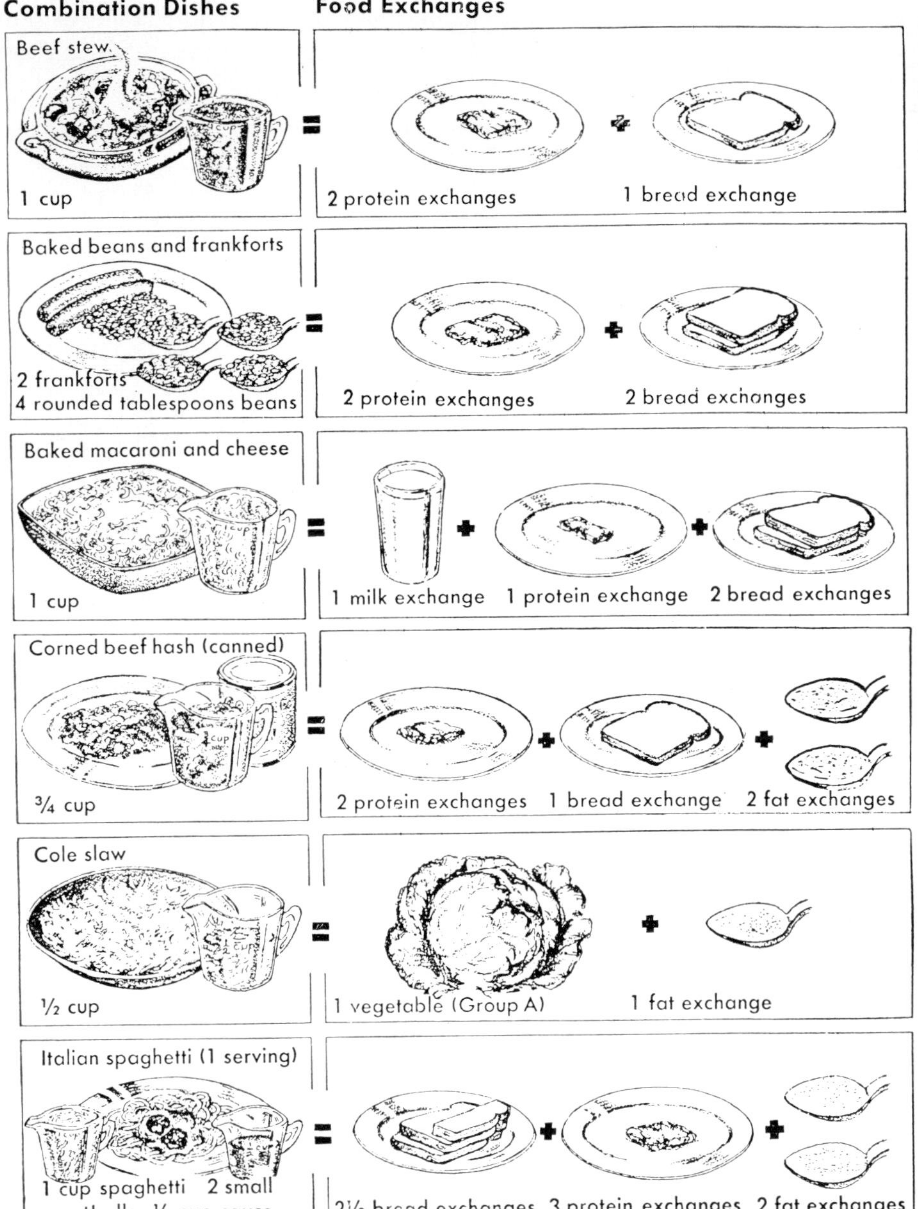

* Exchanges have been computed from figures in U.S. Handbook No. 8. Italian spaghetti computed from a basic recipe.

Exchanges for Combination Dishes*

Each of the following combination dishes may be used, provided that the proper food exchanges are made.

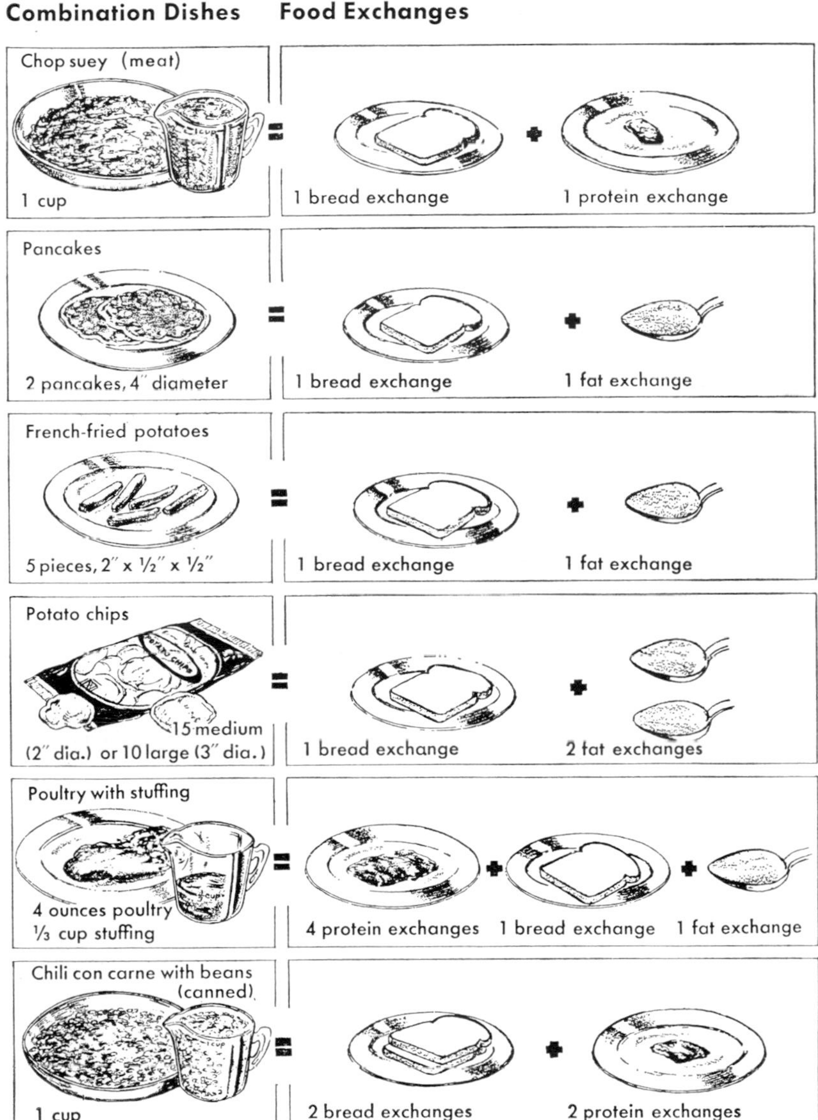

* Exchanges have been computed from figures in U.S. Handbook No. 8.

DESSERT EXCHANGES

In this book, special effort has been made to assure the patient of a normal way of life, and it has been shown how the diabetic diet can closely conform to that of the family. The following discussion concerning desserts has been included as a part of this endeavor.

Although concentrated sweets such as sugar,* frosting, syrups and the like are not allowed, there are desserts which can be used, provided that the proper exchanges for their ingredients are made in the diet. One such dessert is strawberry shortcake which is prepared with fruit, biscuit and whipped cream. The exchange for this dessert is made as follows: ½ biscuit equals 1 slice of bread, 2 tablespoons of unsweetened whipped cream equal 1 teaspoon of butter and 13 strawberries equal 1 fruit exchange. Therefore, to make the proper total exchange for strawberry shortcake, the following foods should be deducted from the total daily food allowance: 1 slice of bread, 1 teaspoon of butter and 1 serving of fruit.

By a similar process of exchange, ½ cup of ice cream may be eaten by subtracting 1 slice of bread and 2 teaspoons of butter from the total daily diet. These and other dessert exchanges are listed and illustrated on the pages that follow. It is intended that, used discretely, these exchanges will help the patient feel less restriction in his diet.

Except when the term unsweetened is used, the exchange values for the following desserts are for regular sweetened desserts and not for artificially sweetened "dietetic" products. This statement applies to desserts such as plain, angel and sponge cakes, cookies, custard and ice cream.

* See discussion of sweetening agents, page 68.

Dessert Exchanges

Certain desserts may be included in the diet, provided that the proper food exchanges are made. The following list shows the desserts and their food exchanges.

Desserts	Food Exchanges
Cake	
Angel or sponge, 1/10 of average cake	2 slices of bread
Plain, 3″×2″×1¾″	2 slices of bread 1 teaspoon of butter
Cookies, plain, 1, 3″ diameter	1 slice of bread
Custard, 1 serving (½ cup)	1½ slices of bread 1 egg
Fruit gelatin, unsweetened (using 1 serving fruit and ½ cup fruit juice)	2 servings of fruit
Fruit shortcake, 1 serving with 2 tablespoons unsweetened whipped cream	1 serving of fruit 1 slice of bread 1 teaspoon of butter
Ice cream, plain, ½ cup	1 slice of bread 2 teaspoons of butter
Plain gelatin (using ½ cup fruit juice)	1 serving of fruit

Dessert Exchanges

Each of the following desserts may be used, provided that the proper food exchanges are made.

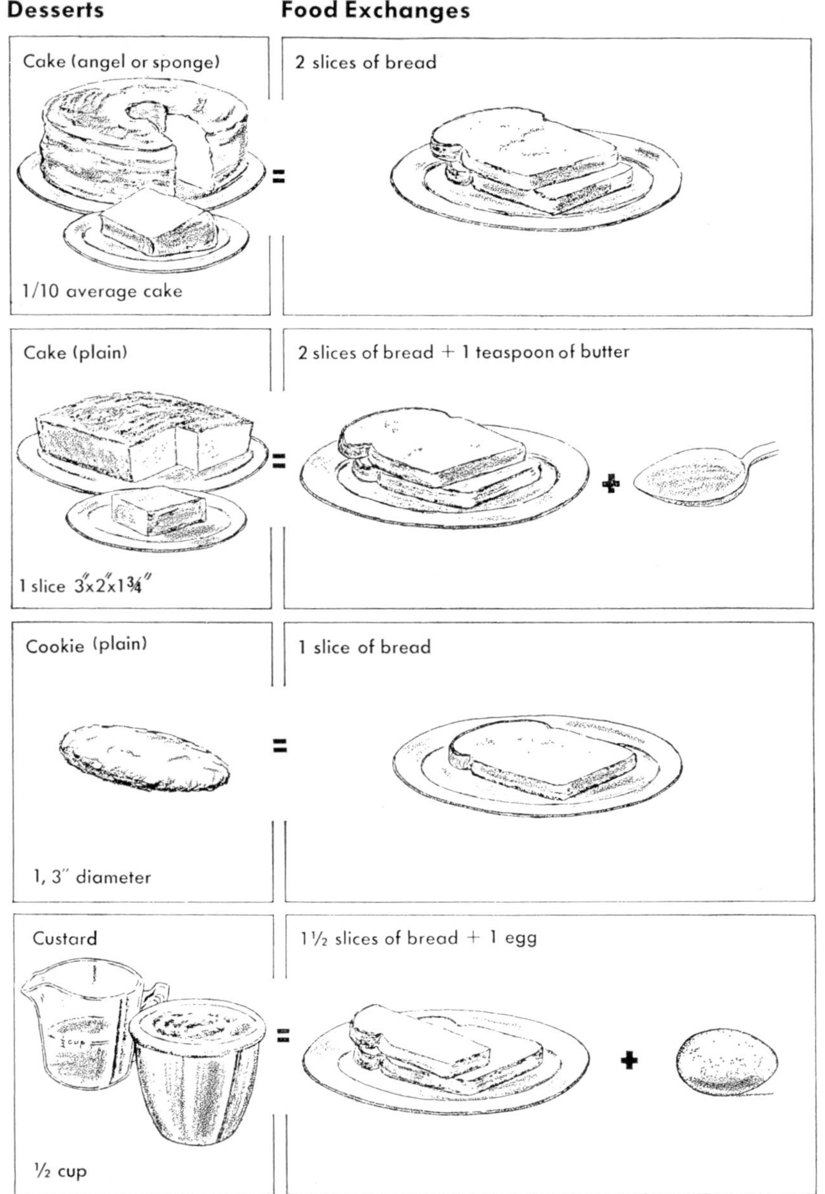

Dessert Exchanges

Each of the following desserts may be used, provided that the proper food exchanges are made.

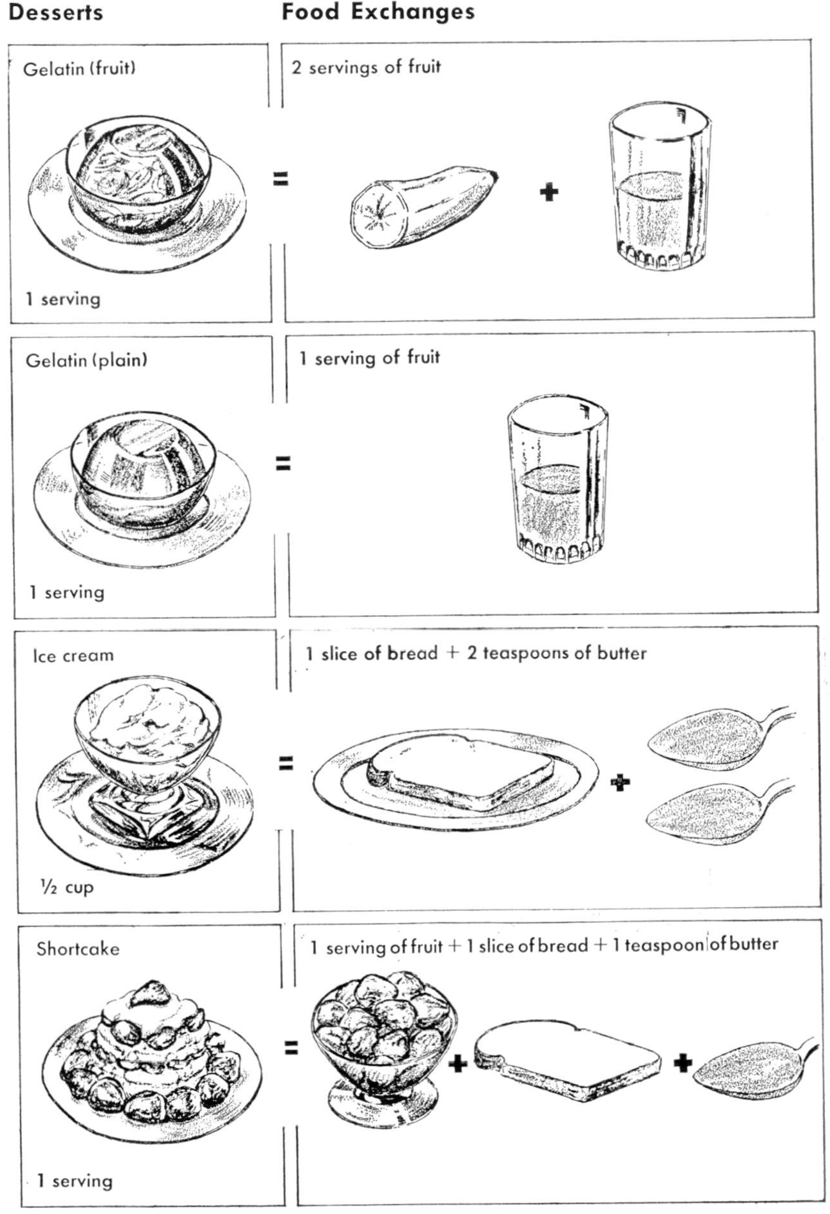

Southern Missionary College
Division Of Nursing, Library
711 Lake Estelle Drive
Orlando, Florida 32803

UNRESTRICTED SEASONINGS AND FOODS

Seasonings and food which contain no appreciable amounts of carbohydrate, protein and fat may be used as desired unless their use is restricted by the presence of conditions other than diabetes.

Seasonings

Allspice
Angostura bitters
Anise
Basil
Bay leaf
Caraway seed
Catsup
Celery
Celery salt
Celery seed
Chervil
Chili powder
Chives
Cinnamon
Cloves
Curry powder
Dill
Garlic
Garlic salt
Ginger
Leeks
Lemon rind
Mace
Marjoram
Mint
Mustard
Nutmeg
Onion juice
Onion salt
Orange rind
Oregano
Parsley
Pepper
Poppy seeds
Poultry seasoning
Rosemary
Saffron
Sage
Sauces, bottled (without sugar)
Tabasco
Tarragon
Thyme
Vanilla extract
Vinegar

Beverages and Soups

Broth (clear)
Bouillon
Coffee
Consommé
Dietetic soft drinks (sugar-free tonic or "pop")
Tea
Tomato juice
Tomato soup (clear)
Vegetable juice
Water (plain or carbonated)

Miscellaneous

Gelatin, dietetic or plain
Pickles, dill or sour
Sugar substitutes*

* See "Sweetening Agents," page 68.

CALCULATION OF THE DIABETIC DIET

The calculation of the diet is not complicated and with the use of simple arithmetic should be accomplished without difficulty. The amounts of the carbohydrate, the protein and the fat in the various foods in the diet can be obtained from the lists of food exchanges or the illustration sheets. Then these totals can be compared with the diet prescription.

Since many foods contain more than one food nutrient, the total carbohydrate is computed by adding the carbohydrate shown on the food exchange lists for dairy products, fruits, group B vegetables, bread, soups, combination dishes and desserts.

The total protein is figured by adding the amounts of protein shown on the exchange lists of dairy products, protein foods, group B vegetables, bread, soups, combination dishes and desserts.

Similarly, the amount of fat contained in dairy products, in protein and fat foods, as well as in soups, combination dishes and desserts are added to obtain the total fat intake for the day.

Then, the sums of the total grams of carbohydrate and protein are multiplied by 4, and the sum of the grams of fat is multiplied by 9, to obtain the calories derived from the 3 food nutrients. Finally, these results are added to obtain the total number of calories in the diet.

The 2 examples of diabetic diets that follow demonstrate the calculation of the diet and also the possibilities offered in selection and combinations of food to fulfill the diet prescription (Tables 6 and 7).

Table 6. Calculation of a Sample Diabetic Diet*

Diet Prescription: Carbohydrate — 150 Grams
Protein — 70 Grams
Fat — 70 Grams
Calories — 1,500

Food	Daily Amount	Grams		
		Carbo-hydrate	Protein	Fat
Milk, whole	2 glasses (1 pint)	24	16	20
Cheese, American	1 ounce	..	8	10
Egg	1	..	7	5
Meat, fish or poultry	4 ounces	..	28	20
Butter or other fat	3 teaspoons	..	..	15
Fruit	4 servings	40	..	..
Vegetables, Group A	Unlimited	..	..	..
Group B	1 serving	10	2	..
Bread	5 slices	75	10	..
Tea or Coffee	Unrestricted	..	..	..
Clear Broth	Unrestricted	..	..	..
	Totals:	149	71	70

Total Carbohydrate	149 grams x 4 calories per gram =	596 calories
Total Protein	71 grams x 4 calories per gram =	284 calories
Total Fat	70 grams x 9 calories per gram =	630 calories
	Total =	1,510 calories

* The figures for the food calculations have been taken from the Food Exchange lists (pp. 27 to 59).

TABLE 7. CALCULATION OF A SAMPLE DIABETIC DIET*

Diet Prescription: Carbohydrate — 150 Grams
Protein — 70 Grams
Fat — 70 Grams
Calories — 1,500

Food	Daily Amount	Grams: Carbo-hydrate	Protein	Fat
Milk, whole	1 glass (8 ounces)	12	8	10
Cheese, American	1 ounce	..	8	10
Egg	1	..	7	5
Meat, fish or poultry	5 ounces	..	35	25
Butter or other fat	4 teaspoons	..	..	20
Fruit	5 servings	50	..	..
Vegetables, Group A	Unlimited	..	..	..
Group B	1 serving	10	2	..
Potato	1 small	15	2	..
Cereal	1 serving	15	2	..
Bread	3 slices	45	6	..
Tea or Coffee	Unrestricted	..	..	..
Clear Broth	Unrestricted	..	..	..
	Totals:	147	70	70

Total Carbohydrate	147 grams x 4 calories per gram =	588 calories
Total Protein	70 grams x 4 calories per gram =	280 calories
Total Fat	70 grams x 9 calories per gram =	630 calories
	Total =	1,498 calories

* The figures for the food calculations have been taken from the Food Exchange lists (pp. 27 to 59).

THE MEAL PLAN

Care is necessary in dividing the total amount of food allowed for the day into meals, since the distribution of food throughout the day is as important as the amount consumed. The division of the total food allowance into meals and intermediate feedings is dependent upon the treatment and the needs determined by the physician.

As a rule, when diet alone is required, the total daily food allowance is divided into approximately 3 equal parts, spaced from 5 to 6 hours apart. There are times when small intermediate feedings are recommended between meals or at bedtime to spread the food intake throughout the day and the evening, thus lessening the amount consumed at any one time.

When insulin therapy is required, intermediate feedings usually are necessary in addition to the 3 regular meals. The number of these supplementary feedings and the hours at which they are needed are set by the physician, since they are an important part of the treatment. This subject is discussed in detail in the chapter dealing with insulin on page 87.

When oral hypoglycemic agents are used, the division of the total food in the diet should be arranged in meals to provide an equal distribution of carbohydrate throughout the day. The number of intermediate feedings and the times when they are to be taken are an individual matter determined by the physician.

Generally, the amount of food to be eaten at any one meal and the time of the meal is a matter of adjustment for the individual patient. Therefore, the following division of food in the daily diet is only a suggested meal plan. This can be rearranged to suit the individual's needs, with attention to food habits and particular tastes.

SAMPLE MEAL PLAN

Morning Meal

Fruit as listed under Carbohydrate Exchanges (p. 39).
Bread, cereal or other foods as listed under Carbohydrate Exchanges (p. 46).
Egg, or other foods chosen from the list of Protein Exchanges (p. 31).
Butter, cream or other foods as listed under Fat Exchanges (p. 35).
Beverage allowed in the diet.
(No sugar or concentrated sweets.)

Noon and Night Meal

Clear broth, as desired. Other soups with regard to their food values (p. 51).
Meat, fish, poultry or other foods under Protein Exchanges (p. 31).
Vegetables as listed under Carbohydrate Exchanges (p. 43).
Bread, cereal, potato or other foods under Carbohydrate Exchanges (p. 46).
Butter, cream or other foods as listed under Fat Exchanges (p. 35).
Beverage allowed in the diet.
Dessert. Fruit as listed under Carbohydrate Exchanges (p. 39) or dessert as listed under Dessert Exchanges (p. 57).
(No sugar or concentrated sweets.)

Intermediate Feedings

Dependent upon the individual needs as prescribed by the physician.

MEAL PLANS FOR SAMPLE DIABETIC DIETS

In order to give the patient some specific ideas for dividing the total food for the day into meals, the sample diabetic diets on pp. 62 and 63 have been used as examples of how this division may be accomplished. In the first column, the foods have been listed in terms of the exchanges. The second column suggests particular foods which may be selected from the various exchange lists.

Each plan is only one of many into which the sample diets could be divided. How the individual will plan his meals is dependent on many factors, including where each meal is eaten—at home, at work or in a restaurant, at what time of the day a hot or cold meal is most enjoyed and whether the patient lives alone or with others. Also, the foods selected from the exchange lists are only a few of the many that may be chosen in order to increase the appeal of the diet.

MEAL PLANS FOR SAMPLE DIABETIC DIETS

I. Meal Plan in Exchanges	Suggested Selections from Exchange Lists
Morning Meal	
1 Fruit Exchange	1 serving Fruit Juice *or* Fruit
1 Protein Exchange	1 Egg
1 Bread Exchange	1 slice Toast with
1 Fat Exchange	1 teaspoon Butter *or* Margarine
Beverage	Clear Coffee
Noon Meal	
	Sandwich made of
2 Protein Exchanges	2 ounces Meat
2 Bread Exchanges	2 slices Bread
1 Fat Exchange	1 teaspoon Butter *or* 1 full teaspoon Mayonnaise
Group A Vegetable, unlimited	Raw Vegetable—Celery Sticks, etc.
1 Fruit Exchange	1 serving Raw Fruit
1 Whole Milk Exchange	1 glass (8 ounces) Whole Milk
Night Meal	
Clear Broth, unlimited	Clear Broth
3 Protein Exchanges	3 ounces Meat, Fish *or* Poultry
1 Bread Exchange	1 serving Rice, Macaroni *or* Potato
1 Group B Vegetable Exchange	1 serving Group B Vegetable
Group A Vegetable, unlimited	Salad with
1 Fat Exchange	1 tablespoon French Dressing
2 Fruit Exchanges	1 double serving Fruit
Beverage	Clear Coffee *or* Tea, with or without Lemon
Intermediate Feeding*	
1 Whole Milk Exchange	1 cup (8 ounces) Whole Milk
1 Bread Exchange	1 serving Crackers

* Intermediate feedings are dependent upon individual needs as prescribed by the physician.

MEAL PLANS FOR SAMPLE DIABETIC DIETS

II. Meal Plan in Exchanges	Suggested Selections from Exchange Lists

Morning Meal

1 Fruit Exchange	1 serving Fruit Juice *or* Fruit
1 Protein Exchange	1 Egg
1 Fat Exchange	1 full strip Bacon
1 Bread Exchange	1 serving Cereal with
½ Whole Milk Exchange	½ cup (4 ounces) Whole Milk
Beverage	Clear Coffee

Noon Meal

Group A Vegetable, unlimited	Tomato Juice
4 Protein Exchanges	4 ounces Meat, Fish *or* Poultry
1 Bread Exchange	1 small Potato
1 Bread Exchange	1 slice Bread with
1 Fat Exchange	1 teaspoon Butter *or* Margarine
1 Group B Vegetable Exchange	1 serving Group B Vegetable
1 Fruit Exchange	1 serving Fruit
Beverage	Clear Coffee *or* Tea, with or without Lemon

Night Meal

Clear Broth, unlimited	Clear Broth
1 Protein Exchange	¼ cup flaked Tuna, Crab *or* Lobster
2 Fat Exchanges	2 full teaspoons Mayonnaise
2 Bread Exchanges	1 Muffin
Group A Vegetables, unlimited	Lettuce and Cucumber
2 Fruit Exchanges	Fruit Gelatin
½ Whole Milk Exchange	½ glass (4 ounces) Whole Milk

Intermediate Feeding*

1 Protein Exchange	1 ounce Cheese
1 Fruit Exchange	1 serving Fruit

* Intermediate feedings are dependent upon individual needs as prescribed by the physician.

CONCENTRATED SWEETS

The term "concentrated sweets" refers to foods such as sugar, honey, marmalade, jam, conserve, frosting, candy, Jello and carbonated beverages. These foods contain carbohydrate and little or none of the other food nutrients. For this reason they have often been termed one-sided foods and are suppliers of empty calories (p. 16).

Concentrated sweets, undesirable for many reasons, are not recommended for the diabetic patient. They are absorbed rapidly and might easily disturb the control of the diabetes as they enter the blood stream quickly. Concentrated sweets replace the more essential foods which are necessary in furnishing adequate mineral and vitamin content to the diet. In addition, it is generally agreed that adjustment to the diabetic diet will result more easily and within a shorter period of time when concerted effort is made to discourage the taste for sweets. When they are omitted there is a lessening of the desire for them.

In addition to concentrated sweets, certain desserts are not recommended for the diabetic patient. These include such foods as pies and pastries containing large amounts of carbohydrate as well as fat, with a correspondingly high caloric content. Thus, these desserts are not included in the dessert exchange list and illustration sheets (pp. 57 to 59).

SWEETENING AGENTS

There are available today several commercial sweetening agents made either from saccharin or sodium (or calcium*) cyclamate. These products have no caloric value and are harmless to the body. Sweetening agents can be purchased in tablet, liquid or granule form which taste quite similar to sugar. For some people they provide needed satisfaction, but for others there is a bitter or metallic after-taste which prevents acceptance of these products. The decision regarding the use of sweetening agents is one which rests with the patient.

However, it should be remembered that the diabetic diet must be followed all one's life, and since this is accomplished more easily when the desire for "sweets" disappears, the use of sweetening agents is not encouraged. A familiar example is a person stopping the use of sugar in coffee. At first the coffee is not satisfying, but within a short time the individual could not be persuaded to add sugar to his coffee. So it is with the diabetic patient. When he learns early to do without sweet flavor in foods and beverages, he will come to enjoy unsweetened foods and as a matter of fact might even develop a distaste for sweets.

* For use in diets restricted in sodium.

DIETETIC FOODS

Many grocery stores assign shelf space for "dietetic" or "special" foods. Although these products are not essential for the diabetic diet, there are some which help in varying the diet, especially water-packed fruit and also gelatin or prepared pudding mixes to which artificial sweetening has been added. Gelatin desserts of this type have little food value because they are usually prepared with water and, therefore, may be used as desired. Pudding mixes that are artificially sweetened have little food value in themselves, but, when prepared with milk, the amount used must be considered as part of the milk allowance of the diet.

Another artificially sweetened product which may help vary the diabetic diet is the group of special dietary drinks, either plain or carbonated. Because of their low food value, they, too, may be used in unlimited amounts.

Special dietetic foods such as breads, crackers, cereals and cereal products need not be used, for although the content of carbohydrate may be lower in many of these, the protein is often increased. Since about 60% of the protein is converted into sugar in the body, there really is little advantage, if any, in their use. "Protein bread" and "Special formula bread" are examples of such products. Also, the claim of less calories per slice of bread is often based only on the fact that the slice of bread is thinner than regularly sliced bread.

Special "nonfattening" or "low calorie" oils, mayonnaise and salad dressings are often made with mineral oil. These products are not recommended, as mineral oil is completely indigestible and, in addition, when used in appreciable amounts, tends to interfere with the proper absorption of certain vitamins in the body.

In many instances, the cost of "dietetic" or "special" foods is more than that of similar regular products. However, the final decision concerning their purchase rests with the patient.

FOOD FADS

Separating facts from fallacies is a necessity and a responsibility of the diabetic patient in order to avoid unnecessary trouble. False claims and food faddism reach into every home through advertising, door-to-door salesmen, magazine articles and lectures. Unless a person is forewarned and forearmed he may become a prey to this misleading information.

The Food and Drug Administration has been seriously concerned with this problem and has done much to prosecute violation of food and drug laws. Still new products appear on the market which, either directly or by inference, claim to be of value in preventing or curing a disease. In reality they are most ineffective for this purpose and may be considered dangerous when one neglects proper medical treatment in the hope that, through some "capsule" or the like, one will find a cure. A survey made by the American Diabetes Association indicates that there are more than 100 food fads and fantasies in circulation today. Therefore, it is an unwise patient who takes chances with his diabetes by trying anything which has not been approved by his physician.

Food faddism presents such a warning picture, since it is difficult for the layman to differentiate between truth and half-truth in regard to food practices. Advertising which uses such phrases as "no sugar added," "no fat added," "low calorie," "dietetic" and various others requires careful scrutinizing and evaluation by the patient. For example, a bread which is labeled "no sugar added" has little advantage, if any, over the standard breads, since all breads are made of some flour and therefore contain carbohydrate regardless of whether or not sugar has been used in the preparation.

Sugar comes in many forms. Sucrose is the granulated sugar familiar to all. The public has often been fooled by products misbranded "no sugar added," by which it is meant, "no sucrose added," and a closer look at the fine print will disclose that other sugars such as honey or molasses or dextrose have been used.

Special dietetic candies present another example of labeling which can be open to misinterpretation. They may be rightly labeled as containing no sugar, yet they do contain fat, skim milk powder and other ingredients which contain calories and should not be added to restricted diets.

Space does not permit a complete dissertation on the volume of products which come under the heading of being "misleading." The diabetic patient is urged to seek authoritative information from his physician, such organizations as the American Diabetes Association* and the American Medical Association,† who will send instructive material upon request, and Government agencies such as the Food and Drug Administration. There is still no question that the best way to obtain the essential food nutrients in the diet is through the use of the protective foods—milk, eggs, meat, fish, poultry, fruits, vegetables and enriched or whole-grain breads and cereals.

* American Diabetes Association, Inc., 18 East 48th Street, New York, N. Y. 10017.

† American Medical Association, 535 North Dearborn Street, Chicago, Illinois 60610.

ALCOHOLIC DRINKS

Drinks containing alcohol should not be taken without permission from the physician.

The objectives of diabetic treatment today, upon which most authorities agree, are the comfort and the contentment of the patient as well as the control of the condition. Through the years, alcoholic beverages have been associated with tradition and hospitality, irrespective of nationality, social status and economic level. As it is the custom for the French and the Italians to take wine with meals, other national and religious groups use wine or other alcoholic beverages when celebrating their holidays or observing their Holy Day traditions.

The use of alcoholic drinks by the person with diabetes requires careful consideration for several reasons. Alcohol is absorbed very rapidly in the body, and each cubic centimeter of pure alcohol furnishes about 7 calories. This source of quick energy not only spares the utilization of food but adds to the total caloric intake as well.

Alcoholic beverages, especially when taken in excess, can easily weaken one's self-control and produce serious consequences. The diabetic control might be disrupted with excessive intake of food. On the other hand, insulin reactions might be precipitated by the delay or the omission of a meal. These conditions might not be readily recognized or could be mistaken for intoxication. In either situation there is a possibility that necessary treatment might not be instituted, with serious complications resulting. The patient with diabetes should not drink alone or in excess and should not substitute alcoholic drinks for regular food intake.

A peculiar reaction may occur in a small percentage of persons taking sulfonylurea compounds. This reaction may occur within minutes after the ingestion of even a small amount of an alcoholic beverage and can last for as long as an hour or more. The usual symptoms include a feeling of warmth, with "flushing" of the face, and/or a throbbing headache, nausea, giddiness, shortness of breath and fast heart beat. Photosensitivity reactions (sensitivity to light) may also occur.

Alcoholic beverages can be classified in 2 groups. One contains no carbohydrate and the other contains carbohydrate in addition to alcohol. The first group includes whiskeys (bourbon, Irish, rye and Scotch), gin, rum and certain brandies with no sugar content. Carbohydrate is contained in varying amounts in liqueurs, wines, malt liquors (such as beer and ale), cider and certain mixed drinks.

The energy and food values supplied by alcoholic beverages must be figured when used by the diabetic patient (see Appendix, p. 209).

Although it would be wise for the diabetic patient to refrain from the use of alcoholic drinks, there probably would be little objection to one "before dinner drink" when taken at home or when attending a dinner or social function with family or friends who know about his diabetic condition. *There should be no drinking under any other circumstances.*

The final decision concerning use of alcoholic drinks rests with the physician after careful consideration of his patient.

DIETS FOR DIABETES AND OTHER CONDITIONS

The diabetic diet can be adjusted to meet the dietary needs of other associated conditions. All diet adjustments must fulfill the diabetic food prescription, but the kinds and the amounts of the foods can be so modified as to be suitable for both the diabetes and the coexistent condition.

On the following pages are included suggestions for altering the sample diabetic diet to meet the requirements of certain conditions. It will be noted that the amounts of carbohydrate, protein and fat still meet the same dietary prescription as the sample adult diabetic diet (p. 62). In some cases foods have been exchanged for other kinds having equal value. In other instances the diets have been modified in texture, sodium content or amounts of certain foods.

The variations of the diabetic diet that have been included are as follows: Sodium Restricted Diets (500 and 1,000 milligrams sodium), Bland Diet, Low Residue Diet, Full Liquid Diet and a discussion of the diet where there are food intolerances.

DIABETIC DIET ADJUSTED FOR SODIUM RESTRICTION

When a mild restriction of sodium is required, it may be necessary to omit only the use of salt at the table and in the preparation of food. When the sodium prescription in the diet is markedly reduced, certain foods that contain large amounts of sodium must be restricted or eliminated. There are available a number of salt substitutes which can be used (with the physician's permission) to add flavor to food and thus make it more palatable.

Two sample diets are presented on the following pages, together with lists of food restrictions. One of these contains 1,000 milligrams of sodium, and the other contains 500 milligrams of sodium. There may need to be further modification of these diets, dependent upon the individual diet prescription. This is always determined by the physician.

DIABETIC DIET ADJUSTED FOR SODIUM RESTRICTION

TABLE 8. SAMPLE DIABETIC DIET CONTAINING 1,000 MILLIGRAMS OF SODIUM

			Grams			Milli-grams
Food	Daily Amount	Modifications of Foods Allowed	Carbo-hydrate	Protein	Fat	Sodium
Milk, whole‡	2 glasses (1 pint)	Regular or homogenized; evaporated, dried or skimmed	24	16	20	240
Egg	1	Cooked without salt	..	7	5	65
Meat, fish or poultry	5 ounces	Fresh meat such as beef, lamb, pork, veal, liver; fresh fish; fresh or frozen poultry (see p. 75 for restrictions)	..	35	25	125
Butter, sweet	4 teaspoons	Oil or low sodium margarine may be exchanged for sweet butter.	..	..	20	4
Fruit	4 servings	Fresh, dried or dietetic canned (see p. 75 for restrictions)	40	..	..	4
Vegetables						
Group A	As desired	Fresh, frozen or dietetic canned such as asparagus, green or wax beans, cabbage, cauliflower, tomato, lettuce, squash and others (see p. 75 for restrictions)	..	..	..	10
Group B	1 serving		10	2	..	10
Potato, rice or macaroni	1 small serving	Cooked without salt	15	2	..	5
Cereal	1 serving (see p. 47 for size of servings)	Puffed wheat, puffed rice, shredded wheat, shredded Ralston, Muffets or "low sodium" cornflakes and other available "low sodium" cereals. Also most cooked cereals (see p. 75 for restrictions)	15	2	..	2
Bread, regular	3 slices	Crackers (except those with salted tops) and rolls may be exchanged for regular bread (see p. 47 for size of serving)	45	6	..	510
Tea or Coffee	As desired	Prepared without salt	..	..	.	..
		Totals	149	70	70	975
		Total Calories		1,576		

DIABETIC DIET ADJUSTED FOR SODIUM RESTRICTION

Restrictions in the Low Sodium Diet Containing 1,000 Milligrams of Sodium*

ALL PRODUCTS CONTAINING ADDED SALT OR SODIUM, BAKING POWDER† OR SODA.

READ ALL LABELS ON CANNED, FROZEN OR PACKAGED FOODS

Cheese ....All cheese and cheese spreads except those which are especially marked "low sodium‡."

Meat, fish ....Salted or smoked meats such as ham, bacon, bologna, tongue, sausage, frankfurters, dried beef, corned beef and canned meats. Meat extracts such as broth, consommé, gravy, bouillon cubes and meat tenderizers. Fish, salted or smoked, frozen fish fillet, shellfish and canned fish except those marked "no salt added."

Fats ....Salted butter, margarine, mayonnaise, salt pork, bacon fat and peanut butter.

Fruits ....Fruit to which sodium ascorbate, sodium benzoate or sodium sulfite have been added. This can be determined by reading the label.

Vegetables ....Canned vegetables or vegetable juices (except dietetic canned), frozen peas and Lima beans, artichoke, beets, beet greens, carrots, celery, chard, dandelion greens, kale, mustard greens, spinach, white turnip and sauerkraut.

Bread ....No more than the number of slices allowed on the diet.

Crackers ....Crackers which have salt sprinkled on top such as Saltines.

Cereals ....Most ready-to-serve cereals except puffed wheat, puffed rice, shredded wheat, Muffets or cereals marked as "low sodium" such as "low sodium" cornflakes.

Flour Products .....Products made with prepared flour mixes such as pancake mix.

Miscellaneous ......Salted nuts, pretzels, potato chips, salted popcorn, relishes, pickles, prepared horseradish, prepared mustard, Worcestershire sauce, soy sauce, catsup, chili sauce, olives, celery salt, onion salt, garlic salt, rennet tablets, Dutch process cocoa and malted milk.

Salt ....Used either at the table or in cooking.

---

* Adapted from Restrictions on Low Sodium Diet, Frances Stern Nutrition Center, The Boston Dispensary, 1963.

† Low sodium baking powders are available on the market. Labels should be read carefully.

‡ Throughout this book cheese has been suggested as an exchange for milk. However, 1 ounce of cheese contains approximately 200 milligrams of sodium and therefore should be used with a sodium restriction only when advised by the physician.

DIABETIC DIET ADJUSTED FOR SODIUM RESTRICTION

TABLE 9. SAMPLE DIABETIC DIET CONTAINING 500 MILLIGRAMS OF SODIUM

Food	Daily Amount	Modifications of Foods Allowed	Grams: Carbohydrate	Grams: Protein	Grams: Fat	Milligrams: Sodium
Milk, whole‡	2 glasses (1 pint)	Regular or homogenized; evaporated, dried or skimmed	24	16	20	240
Egg	1	Cooked without salt	..	7	5	65
Meat, fish or poultry	5 ounces	Fresh meat such as beef, lamb, pork, veal, liver; fresh fish; fresh or frozen poultry (see p. 77 for restrictions)	..	35	25	125
Butter, sweet	4 teaspoons	Oil or low sodium margarine may be exchanged for sweet butter	..	..	20	4
Fruit	4 servings	Fresh, dried or dietetic canned (see p. 77 for restrictions)	40	..	..	4
Vegetables						
Group A	As desired	Fresh, frozen or dietetic canned such as asparagus, green or wax beans, cabbage, cauliflower, tomato, lettuce, squash and others (see p. 77 for restrictions)	..	.	..	10
Group B	1 serving		10	2	..	10
Potato, rice or macaroni	1 small serving	Cooked without salt	15	2	..	5
Cereal	1 serving (see p. 47 for size of servings)	Puffed wheat, puffed rice, shredded wheat, shredded Ralston, Muffets or "low sodium" cornflakes and other available "low sodium" cereals. Also most cooked cereals (see p. 77 for restrictions)	15	2	..	2
Bread, low sodium	3 slices	*Low sodium bread only.* Low sodium crackers, potato, rice, macaroni or allowed cereals may be exchanged for low sodium bread. (See p. 47 for size of servings.)	45	6	..	30
Tea or Coffee	As desired	Prepared without salt	..	..	..	.
		Totals	149	70	70	495
		Total Calories		1,576		

DIABETIC DIET ADJUSTED FOR SODIUM RESTRICTION

Restrictions in the Low Sodium Diet Containing 500 Milligrams of Sodium*

ALL PRODUCTS CONTAINING ADDED SALT OR SODIUM, BAKING POWDER† OR SODA.

READ ALL LABELS ON CANNED, FROZEN OR PACKAGED FOODS.

Cheese ....All cheese and cheese spreads except those which are especially marked "low sodium‡."

Meat, fish ....Salted or smoked meats such as ham, bacon, bologna, tongue, sausage, frankfurters, dried beef, corned beef and canned meats. Meat extracts such as broth, consommé, gravy, bouillon cubes and meat tenderizers. Fish, salted or smoked, frozen fish fillet, shellfish and canned fish except those marked "no salt added."

Fats ....Salted butter, margarine, mayonnaise, salt pork, bacon fat and peanut butter.

Fruits ....Fruit to which sodium ascorbate, sodium benzoate or sodium sulfite have been added. This can be determined by reading the label.

Vegetables .... Canned vegetables or vegetable juices (except dietetic canned), frozen peas and Lima beans, artichoke, beets, beet greens, carrots, celery, chard, dandelion greens, kale, mustard greens, spinach, white turnip and sauerkraut.

Bread ....All regular bread made with salt.

Crackers ....All regular crackers made with salt.

Cereals ....Most ready-to-serve cereals except puffed wheat, puffed rice, shredded wheat, Muffets or cereals marked as "low sodium."

Flour Products .....Products made with prepared flour mixes such as pancake mix.

Miscellaneous ......Salted nuts, pretzels, potato chips, salted popcorn, relishes, pickles, prepared horseradish, prepared mustard, Worcestershire sauce, soy sauce, catsup, chili sauce, olives, celery salt, onion salt, garlic salt, rennet tablets, Dutch process cocoa and malted milk.

Salt ....Used either at the table or in cooking.

---

* Adapted from Restrictions on Low Sodium Diet, Frances Stern Nutrition Center, The Boston Dispensary, 1963.

† Low sodium baking powders are available on the market. Labels should be read carefully.

‡ Throughout this book cheese has been suggested as an exchange for milk. However, 1 ounce of cheese contains approximately 200 milligrams of sodium and therefore should be used with a sodium restriction only when prescribed by the physician.

DIABETIC AND BLAND DIET

TABLE 10. SAMPLE DIABETIC AND BLAND DIET

Food	Daily Amount	Modifications of Foods Allowed	Grams: Carbohydrate	Grams: Protein	Grams: Fat
Milk, whole	2 glasses (1 pint)	Regular or homogenized; evaporated, dried or skimmed. Use at room temperature as beverage, on cereal or in cooking	24	16	20
Cheese	1 ounce	Mild white or yellow cheese such as American cheddar or cottage (see p. 79 for restrictions)	..	8	10
Egg	1	Baked, boiled, poached or scrambled in double boiler	..	7	5
Meat, fish or poultry	4 ounces	Tender meats such as beef, lamb, veal, liver; white fish such as haddock, cod, halibut; chicken or turkey. Baked, boiled, broiled or roasted. (See p. 79 for restrictions)	..	28	20
Butter or margarine	3 teaspoons	Cream, cream cheese or oil may be used as an exchange (see p. 79 for restrictions)	..	..	15
Fruit	3 servings	Diluted orange, grapefruit or other strained juices; ripe banana, dietetic canned pears, peaches, applesauce or cooked fruit, with skin and seeds removed (see p. 79 for restrictions)	30	..	..
Vegetables					
Group A	As desired	Tender cooked vegetables such as green beans, carrots, beets, asparagus tips, squash and young greens; vegetable juices (see p. 79 for restrictions)	..	..	..
Group B	1 serving		10	2	..
Bread or exchanges	6 servings	White or light rye bread or crackers; refined white cereals such as cream of wheat, farina, cornflakes, puffed wheat or puffed rice; potato, macaroni, noodles, spaghetti or white rice (see p. 79 for restrictions)	90	12	..
		Totals	154	73	70
		Total Calories		1,538	

DIABETIC AND BLAND DIET

A bland diet contains most of the foods in the diabetic diet, with a few exceptions. The foods must be bland, nonirritating and nonstimulating to the digestive tract, and neither too hot nor too cold. Certain meats, fruits, vegetables and whole grains are not used, since they contain cellulose or roughage which is not usually permitted. *Since there are various opinions, based on individual experience with patients, of foods to be retained or omitted in the bland diet, the following outline is a suggested sample which may be modified by the physician.*

Restrictions in the Bland Diet

Milk ....Hot or very cold.

Cheese ....Any cheese or cheese spread containing spices, onion, chives, pimento or pineapple or the so-called "strong cheeses."

Egg ....Fried.

Meat and fish ......Meats containing long fibers which require long cooking; smoked or pickled meats and fish such as ham, corned beef and herring; spiced or prepared meats such as sausage, frankfurters, bologna and liverwurst; meat broths, extractives and gravies.

Fats ....Seasoned oils such as French dressing, mayonnaise and salad dressing; lard, salt pork and bacon fat; and olives and nuts.

Fruits ....All raw fruits except banana and strained, diluted juices. Fruits with skins, seeds or fiber such as berries, cherries, cranberries, dates, figs, grapes, pineapple, plums, raisins and rhubarb.

Vegetables ....Artichokes, broccoli, Brussels sprouts, cabbage, cauliflower, celery, cucumber, green and red pepper, okra, onions, parsnips, radishes, sauerkraut, tomatoes and turnip; baked beans, corn, dried peas and beans and Lima beans.

Bread ....Coarse breads such as those containing whole wheat, bran or seeds.

Crackers ....Crackers containing whole wheat, bran or seeds or those fried in deep fat.

Cereals ....Cereals containing bran, whole grain cereals or whole grain rice.

Miscellaneous ......Condiments such as pepper, mustard, catsup, relishes, pickles, horseradish, Worcestershire sauce and chili sauce; most spices, vinegar, popcorn, potato chips and fried foods.

Beverages ....Coffee, sometimes tea, carbonated beverages, alcoholic beverages, cocoa and hot chocolate.

DIABETIC AND LOW RESIDUE DIET

TABLE 11. SAMPLE DIABETIC AND LOW RESIDUE DIET

Food	Daily Amount	Modifications of Foods Allowed	Grams Carbohydrate	Grams Protein	Grams Fat
Milk, whole	2 glasses (1 pint)	Regular or homogenized; evaporated, dried or skimmed. Use at room temperature as beverage, on cereal or in cooking. Milk may or may not be boiled	24	16	20
Cheese	1 ounce	Mild white or yellow cheese such as American cheddar or cottage (see p. 81 for restrictions)	..	8	10
Egg	1	Baked, boiled, poached or scrambled in double boiler	.	7	5
Meat, fish or poultry	4 ounces	Ground tender meats, such as beef, lamb, veal, liver; white fish such as haddock, cod, halibut; chicken or turkey. Boiled, broiled or baked (see p. 81 for restrictions)	..	28	20
Butter or margarine	3 teaspoons	Cream, cream cheese or oil may be used as an exchange (see p. 81 for restrictions)	..	..	15
Fruit	3 servings	Diluted orange, grapefruit or other strained juices; ripe banana, dietetic canned pears, peaches, applesauce or cooked fruit with skin and seeds removed (see p. 81 for restrictions)	30	..	..
Vegetables					
Group A	As desired	Cooked, strained, tender vegetables such as green beans, carrots, beets, asparagus tips, squash and young greens; vegetable juices (see p. 81 for restrictions)	..	..	..
Group B	1 serving		10	2	..
Bread or exchanges	6 servings	White or light rye bread or crackers; refined white cereals such as cream of wheat, farina, cornflakes, puffed wheat or puffed rice; potato, macaroni, noodles, spaghetti or white rice (see p. 81 for restrictions)	90	12	..
Tea, Coffee	As desired		..	.	..
Consommé or clear broth	As desired		..	..	..
		Totals	154	73	70
		Total Calories		1,538	

DIABETIC AND LOW RESIDUE DIET

The degree of restriction of the low residue diet will be determined by the physician, since the restriction will depend on the condition for which it is prescribed, as well as the particular individual. The modification of the sample diabetic diet to meet the requirements of a low residue diet is calculated on the preceding page.

Restrictions in the Low Residue Diet

Milk .... In certain cases milk may not be allowed on low residue diets.

Cheese .... Any cheese or cheese spread containing spices, onion, chives, pimento, pineapple or the so-called "strong cheeses." Very low residue diet may require only cottage cheese when tolerated.

Egg .... Fried.

Meat, fish or poultry ... Meats containing long fibers; smoked or pickled meats such as ham and corned beef; spiced or prepared meats such as sausage, frankfurters, bologna and liverwurst; meats which have not been ground; skin of chicken or turkey.

Fats .... Peanut butter and nuts.

Fruits .... All raw fruits except banana and strained juices. Fruits with skins, seeds or fiber such as berries, cherries, cranberries, dates, figs, grapes, melon, pineapple, plums, raisins and rhubarb. Very low residue diets would limit fruit to strained citrus juices.

Vegetables .... All raw, unstrained or gas-forming vegetables except vegetable juices. Artichokes, broccoli, Brussels sprouts, cabbage, cauliflower, celery, cucumber, green and red pepper, okra, onions, parsnips, radishes, sauerkraut, tomatoes and turnip; baked beans, corn, dried peas and beans and Lima beans.

Bread .... All whole grain bread, hot breads and breads containing seeds.

Crackers .... All whole grain crackers, crackers containing seeds or those fried in deep fat.

Cereals .... Whole grain cereals such as whole wheat flakes, cooked whole wheat or oat cereals or whole grain rice.

Flour Products .... Mixes made of whole grain flour such as buckwheat flour or those containing fruits such as blueberry pancake mix.

Miscellaneous .... All fried foods, strong condiments such as pepper, mustard, catsup, relishes, pickles, horseradish, Worcestershire sauce and chili sauce.

Beverages .... Alcoholic beverages usually not allowed. Other beverages dependent upon the condition.

DIABETIC AND FULL LIQUID DIET

Table 12. Sample Diabetic and Full Liquid Diet

Food	Daily Amount	Modifications of Foods Allowed	Grams Carbo-hydrate	Grams Protein	Grams Fat
Milk, whole	4 glasses (1 quart)	Regular or homogenized; evaporated, dried or skimmed. May be used as beverage, on cereal or in cooking	48	32	40
Eggs	4	Used in eggnog or as soft custard. Homogenized meat such as baby beef, veal, liver, pork or chicken may be exchanged for egg and used in soup	..	28	20
Butter or Margarine	2 teaspoons	May be used in soup or in cereal. Cream may be exchanged for butter	..	..	10
Fruit	6 servings	Fruit juices such as orange, grapefruit, tangerine, apple and prune. (See p. 83 for restrictions.)	60	..	.
Vegetables					
Group A	As desired	Puréed vegetables such as green beans, wax beans, carrots, peas, beets, squash, asparagus tips and young greens. Used as juices or in soups. (See p. 83 for restrictions.)	..		..
Group B	1 serving		10	2	..
Cereal	2 servings	Refined white cereals such as cream of wheat, cream of rice, farina and strained oatmeal. Used as gruels. (See p. 83 for restrictions.)	30	4	..
Tea, Coffee	As desired		..	..	..
Consommé or clear broth	As desired		..	..	..
		Totals	148	66	70
		Total Calories		1,486	

DIABETIC AND FULL LIQUID DIET

The liquid diet is usually a temporary one and is always prescribed by the physician. A full liquid diet contains the foods in the regular diabetic diet with the exception of meat, fish, poultry, bread and crackers. Occasionally, meat in the homogenized form will be included in soups. The protein exchanges can be fulfilled by the use of eggs. Fruits can be taken in the form of juice and vegetables can be strained and used in soups. The foods in the bread group can be exchanged for cereals in the form of gruels. The diabetic and full liquid diet is shown on the preceding page.

Restrictions in the Full Liquid Diet

Cheese .... All cheese.

Meat, fish or poultry ... All meat, fish or poultry which cannot be finely homogenized and combined with bouillon or broth or served in soups.

Egg .... Baked, boiled, poached or scrambled.

Fruits .... Whole fruits of any kind.

Vegetables .... Uncooked or cooked whole vegetables.

Bread .... All breads, crackers, potato (except as soup), macaroni products and rice.

Cereals .... Dry cereals and unstrained, cooked whole grain cereal.

FOOD INTOLERANCES

The patient may be sensitive to one or more foods which appear on the diabetic diet list. Sensitivity to a single food should not present any problem, since the lists of food exchanges offer many possibilities for substitution. However, when there is an intolerance involving a large group of foods such as all fruits or many protein foods such as milk, cheese and egg, there may need to be a careful evaluation of the diet with the physician.

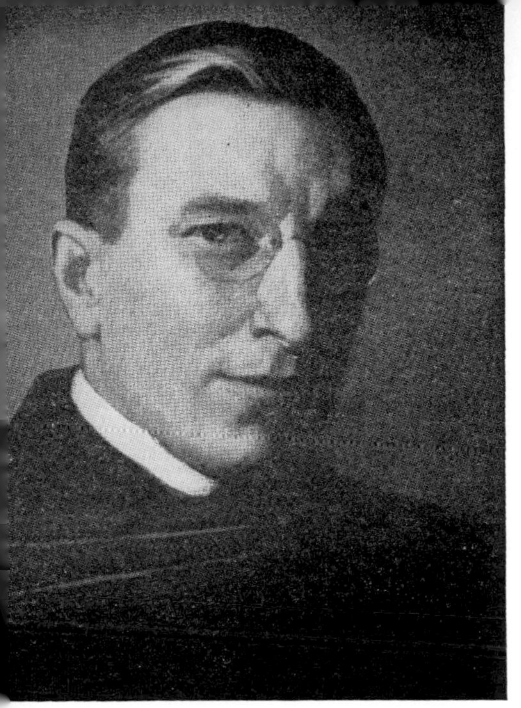

SIR FREDERICK GRANT BANTING
1891–1941

Born in Canada and educated at the University of Toronto. Served in World War I and was awarded the Military Cross. Director of Banting and Best Department of Medical Research, which was founded in the University of Toronto in 1923. Same year received Nobel Prize for discovery of insulin. In 1924 Banting Research Foundation was established, and in 1930 Banting Institute was opened in Toronto. Created Knight of the British Empire in 1934. Elected Fellow of the Royal Society of London, 1935. Killed in airplane accident in Newfoundland in 1941.

BANTING AND BEST, WHOSE DISCOVERY OF INSULIN GAVE DIABETICS THE CHANCE TO LIVE NORMAL, HAPPY AND USEFUL LIVES

DR. CHARLES HERBERT BEST
1899–

Born West Pembroke, Maine (parents Canadians). Educated at University of Toronto and University of London. Served in World War I and was Director of the Royal Canadian Navy Medical Research Division during World War II. Appointed Director, Department of Physiology, University of Toronto, in 1929. Director of Banting and Best Department of Medical Research, in 1941, and in 1953 also appointed Director of the Charles H. Best Institute. Honorary Degrees received from Universities of Chicago, Paris, Cambridge, Amsterdam, Liege, Oxford, Dalhousie, Queens, Chile, Uruguay, San Marcos (Peru), Melbourne, Laval, Maine, Venezuela, Edinburgh, Aristotelian University of Thessaloniki, and Freie University of Berlin. Vice-President of British Diabetic Association since its founding in 1934. American Diabetes Association: President 1948-49; past member of the Council and currently Honorary President; Chairman of the Editorial Board of The Journal of the American Diabetes Association, 1952-58. Elected Honorary Member of the European Association for the Study of Diabetes, 1965. (Ashley and Crippen, Toronto, Can.)

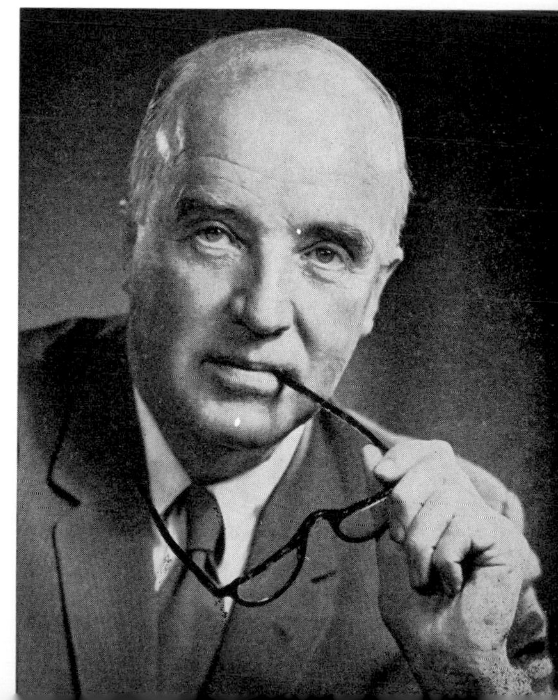

3. INSULIN

The Discovery of insulin in 1921 by Sir Frederick G. Banting and Dr. Charles H. Best was one of the outstanding achievements in medical science. Although a detailed account of the pertinent events that preceded and followed this exciting discovery is not intended in the scope of a book such as this, certain endeavors deserve special mention.

As early as 1869, a German pathologist and anatomist, Langerhans, described the cells (now called islands of Langerhans) in the pancreas from which insulin is derived. During the latter part of the 19th century two German scientists, Minkowski and Von Mering, noted that diabetes could be produced in dogs by the removal of the pancreas. This was the first time that diabetes was produced experimentally. In the years that followed, many investigators tried without success to use products derived from the pancreas in a search for treatment or a cure for diabetes. Then in 1921 Dr. Banting and Dr. Best uncovered the secret of obtaining insulin from the pancreas. The credit for perfecting the insulin for use, by improving the method of its extraction from the pancreas of animals, belongs to Dr. Collip, a Canadian chemist.

For many years, this insulin preparation was used when diet alone was not sufficient for diabetic control. Then, in 1936 Dr. H. Hagedorn of Denmark and his associates found that by adding a protein (protamine) to insulin its action could be prolonged for a period of 12 hours as compared with 4 to 6 hours. Following this, Scott and Fisher at the University of Toronto discovered that, by adding zinc to the protamine insulin, the resultant preparation, protamine-zinc insulin, was effective in controlling blood-sugar levels for a period of 24 hours or longer. For the first time, diabetic control could be achieved in many instances, with one injection of insulin daily instead of multiple injections.

Although protamine-zinc insulin was effective for many, there still were patients who required additional injections of regular insulin for adequate diabetic control. In 1943, as a result of further study, the first of another group of insulin preparations, the so-called intermediate-acting insulins, was developed.

This preparation called globin insulin was followed by two other intermediate-acting insulins, NPH insulin and lente insulin. These insulin preparations, together with rapid-acting insulin (unmodified insulin), and long-acting insulin (protamine-zinc insulin), now permitted a choice of the preparations best suited to the needs of the individual patient.

There is no known substitute for insulin when its use is indicated for treatment. Up to the present time there is no form of *insulin* which, when taken by mouth, is effective in the control of diabetes. In the process of digestion, insulin is changed in the stomach by the digestive juices and loses its value in the treatment of diabetes. The patient should be deeply grateful for the discovery of insulin, as well as encouraged, and comforted by the progress that has been made since its discovery.

Insulin is required when there is not sufficient usable or "free" insulin in the body to use and store the sugar derived from the prescribed diet. The insulin used for this purpose ("bottle insulin") is a liquid preparation obtained from the pancreas of animals. When taken by injection this insulin acts in much the same manner as body insulin and is an effective and neces-

Interdependence of Diet and Insulin

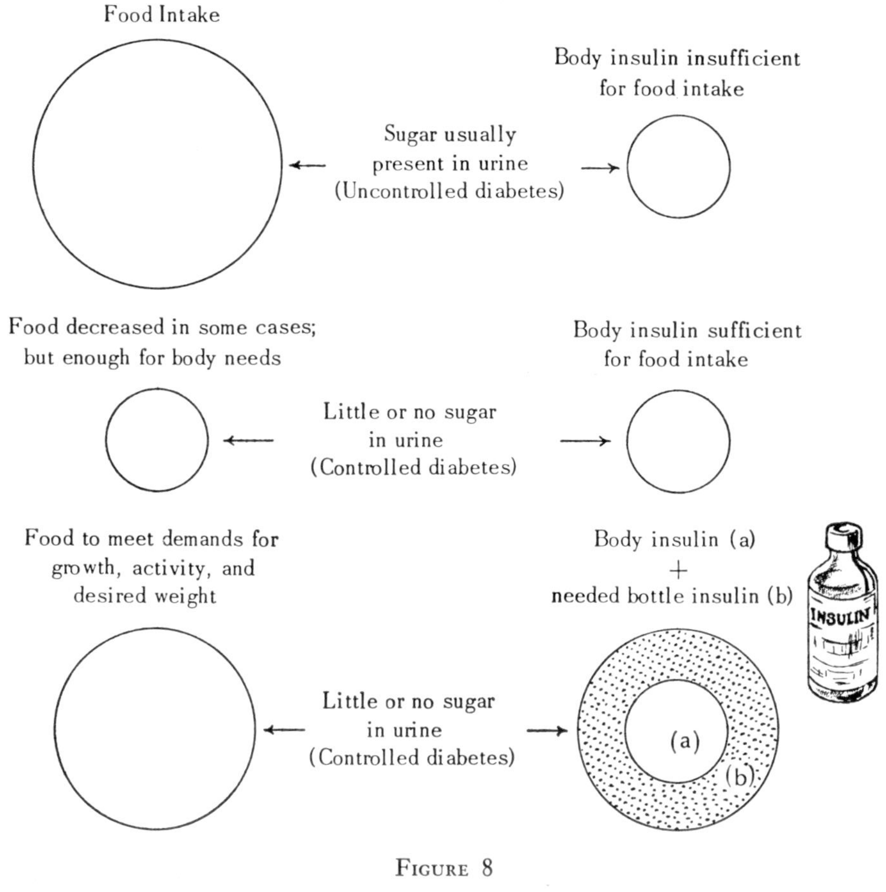

FIGURE 8

sary part of treatment when essential for the control of diabetes (Fig. 8).

Insulin therapy, when indicated, is the most effective means of controlling diabetes in the shortest possible time. The amount of insulin required to achieve good diabetic control often will aid in determining the severity of the diabetes and may give a clue as to whether or not oral drugs can be used successfully at a later date (Chap. 5, Oral Hypoglycemic Agents).

Usually children require insulin therapy. This is most often the case with adolescents and young adults. Many adults require insulin, especially when more liberal diets are necessary to maintain or attain desired weight. Often, when diabetes develops during middle life or later, the need for insulin therapy or oral drugs depends upon the patient's adherence to the prescribed diet as well as upon the severity of the diabetes.

Even though the diabetes is well controlled with oral hypoglycemic agents, occasions may arise when they are no longer effective and treatment with insulin becomes necessary. This may be the case during the course of severe infections or other complications which may alter the severity of the diabetes, temporarily or for longer periods of time. *Therefore, whenever possible, patients should have the technical knowledge and the equipment necessary for the injection of insulin.*

In certain selected cases, the insulin injection procedure may not be feasible. The patient may have physical disabilities such as poor eyesight or arthritis, and there may be no available family members or friends to assume the responsibility for the daily insulin injection. Under such conditions, the use of an oral drug may be prescribed at the outset of treatment, provided that the physician considers the patient to be suitable for this type of therapy.

The kind and the amount of insulin to be used is always determined and prescribed by the physician.

There have been great advances in the development of insulin preparations since insulin was first discovered in 1921. Not only have these preparations facilitated the treatment for both patient and physician, but also they have been the means of achieving better diabetic control during the 24-hour period, and often with fewer daily injections. All insulin preparations are derived from the pancreas of animals, chiefly the cow and the hog. The potency and the stability of these preparations have been determined carefully by approved methods and conform to standards that are established and accepted throughout the world. The chemical formula for insulin is now known and there is the possibility that insulin will be synthesized in the not too distant future.

An adequate supply of insulin should always be available so that the prescribed daily amount is assured. It is wise also to have an extra syringe and needles available. The bottle of insulin should be discarded when there are signs of discoloration or deterioration of the contents. An expiration date is stated on every bottle, and this should be checked so that insulin is not used after the stated date. Insulin should be kept in a cool place, preferably a refrigerator, but freezing should be avoided. However, when desired for convenience, the bottle that is in use may be kept safely at room temperature. Extra supplies of insulin that are kept in reserve require refrigeration. Temperatures, heat and cold, that are too extreme should be avoided, and the bottle of insulin needs to be protected from strong light (sunlight).

All insulin preparations, other than unmodified insulin or regular and globin insulin, must be mixed thoroughly just before use. Vigorous shaking of the bottle is to be avoided. A thoroughly mixed solution is accomplished by rotating the bottle in the palms of the hand and inverting the bottle from end to end. These procedures need to be repeated several times to ensure uniform and constant proportions of the ingredients with each injection (see Procedure for Injection of Insulin, p. 105). Failure to mix insulin solutions correctly can result in irregularity of the effects of the individual doses.

KINDS OF INSULIN PREPARATIONS

There are several insulin preparations. The kind of insulin selected by the physician is intended to meet the special needs of the individual and should not be changed by the patient, unless recommended by the physician.

At the present time the following kinds of insulin are available: insulin (unmodified insulin or regular insulin), protamine zinc insulin (frequently referred to as protamine insulin), globin insulin, NPH insulin and lente insulin, two additional types of which are semilente insulin and ultralente insulin. A description of the various insulin preparations follows.

Rapid-Acting Insulin

Insulin

Insulin, commonly referred to as unmodified insulin or regular insulin, is a water-clear solution made from zinc insulin crystals and is contained in a round bottle. The action is rapid, and its effect is of short duration, lasting from about 5 to 7 hours. The greatest blood-sugar-lowering effect develops about 2 to 3 hours after the injection.

Often insulin is used in conjunction with slow- or intermediate-acting insulin in the form of a mixture (p. 127), or separate injections are prescribed so that better control can be accomplished. Insulin is used also in emergencies such as in the treatment of diabetic acidosis and coma. Often it is used alone or in combination with other insulin preparations during the course of infections, surgery or other acute conditions.

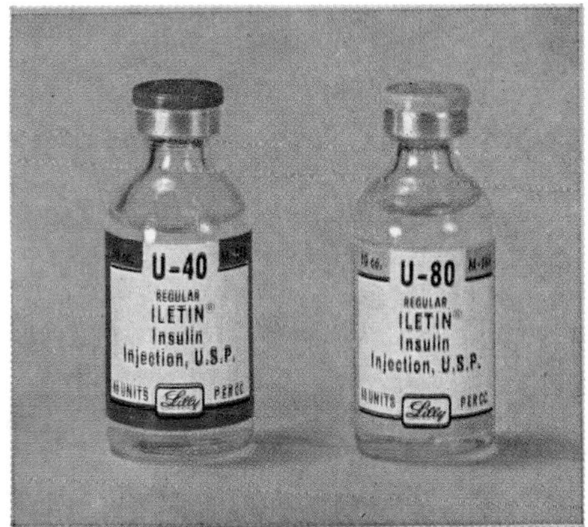

PLATE 1. Insulin (unmodified insulin or regular insulin) for rapid effect. (Eli Lilly & Co.)

Long-Acting Insulin

Protamine Zinc Insulin

Protamine zinc insulin, commonly referred to as protamine insulin, has a cloudy, milky appearance after it has been mixed. It is contained in a round bottle. In addition to insulin, this preparation contains zinc and a protein substance (protamine) which causes it to be absorbed more slowly than regular insulin from the site of injection. The blood-sugar-lowering effect lasts for as long as 36 to 48 hours, and the greatest effect usually develops from about 14 to 20 hours after the injection.

Usually, one daily injection of protamine zinc insulin is sufficient to control most mild or moderately severe diabetes. However, in some instances insulin in addition to protamine zinc insulin is needed to obtain adequate diabetic control. This is accomplished either by means of separate injections of insulin or with the use of insulin mixtures. For these mixtures, a larger amount of insulin than protamine zinc insulin is used. The proportion prescribed most often is 1 part of protamine zinc insulin to 2 parts of insulin (see Insulin Mixtures, p. 127).

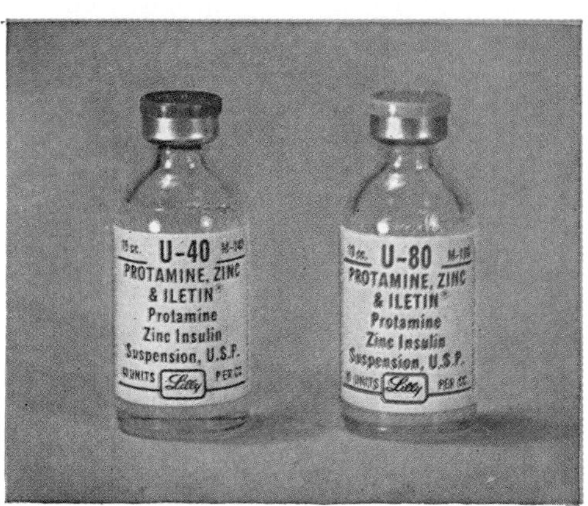

PLATE 2. Protamine zinc insulin for prolonged effect. (Eli Lilly & Co.)

Intermediate-Acting Insulins

In 1936 when protamine zinc insulin was first used, the treatment of diabetes was greatly facilitated. Many patients who previously had required several injections of insulin each day were able to obtain good diabetic control with only one daily injection. However, while the use of protamine zinc insulin resulted in a tremendous advance in treatment, it still did not serve as an ideal preparation for many patients with moderately severe or severe diabetes. With this group, insulin was needed in addition to protamine zinc insulin to obtain the diabetic control desired.

Insulin was taken by separate injections to augment the action of the protamine zinc insulin, or mixtures of protamine zinc insulin and insulin were devised to attain better diabetic control. The technique essential for the preparation of insulin mixtures was rather difficult and required careful instruction to prevent possible errors either in the measurement of the insulins or in the preparation of the mixtures in the syringe.

Often, too, it was difficult to obtain the exact blood-sugar-lowering effect throughout the day and the night without upsetting the patient's mode of living. Rather than readjust this to fit the action of insulin, an attempt was made to produce an insulin preparation to meet the usual needs of the patient.

Thus, the introduction of intermediate-acting insulins followed much study and research—the first globin insulin and, later NPH (Isophane) insulin and lente insulin. With the use of intermediate-acting insulins it was possible, with few exceptions, to prescribe the kind of insulin best suited to the individual patient and thereby maintain the blood-sugar-levels desired throughout the 24-hour period. Also, when more rapid action was needed, insulin could be added to NPH insulin or lente insulin, in the same syringe, without significantly changing the individual actions of each preparation.

On occasion, at the discretion of the physician, intermediate-acting insulin, with or without the addition of regular insulin, may be prescribed in divided doses to achieve better control of the diabetes and to avoid the occurrence of insulin reactions.

A description of the intermediate-acting insulins follows.

Globin Insulin

Globin insulin is a clear, amber-colored solution contained in a round bottle. In addition to insulin this preparation contains globin and zinc. The action of globin insulin lasts up to 24 hours, and the greatest blood-sugar-lowering effect develops about 8 to 16 hours after the injection.

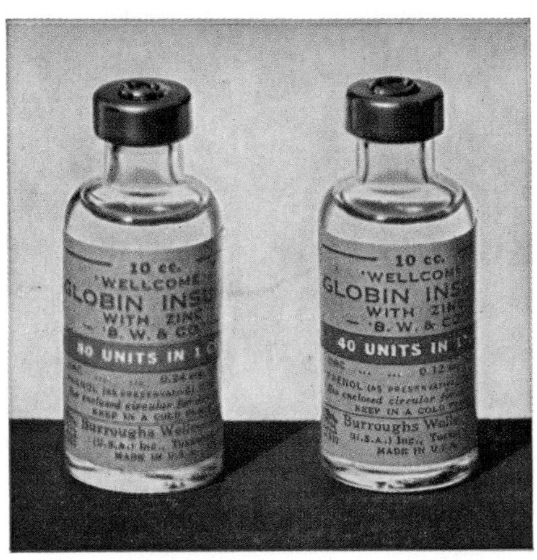

PLATE 3. Globin Insulin for intermediate effect. (Burroughs Wellcome & Co., Inc.)

NPH (Isophane) Insulin

NPH (Isophane) insulin has a cloudy, milky appearance and is contained in square-shaped bottles with blue labels. This insulin consists of a suspension of crystals of insulin together with protamine and zinc. It is necessary that this preparation be mixed thoroughly before it is withdrawn from the bottle so that the proportions of the ingredients are the same for each insulin injection. The blood-sugar-lowering effect of NPH insulin usually lasts 24 to 28 hours, and its greatest effect develops about 8 to 12 hours after the injection.

NPH insulin meets the needs of a large percentage of patients.

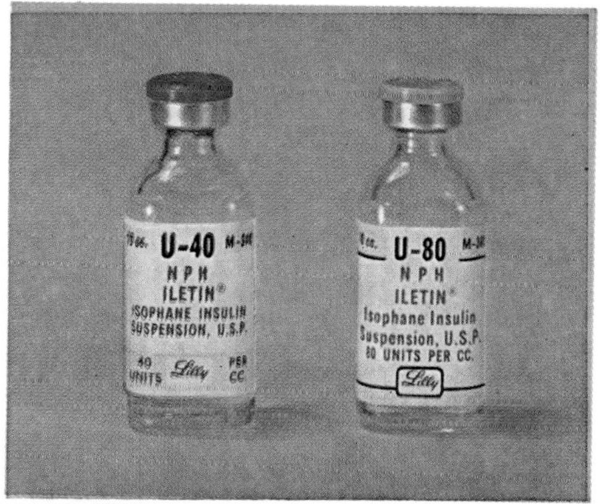

PLATE 4. NPH (Isophane) insulin for intermediate effect. (Eli Lilly & Co.)

Lente Insulin

Lente insulin is a cloudy, milky-appearing solution contained in a round bottle with 6-sided shoulders (Hexanek). A large "L," black striped, is at the left of the colored printing on the label. The action of this preparation is very similar to that of NPH insulin, the difference being in the ingredients. Lente insulin contains only insulin and zinc. As with NPH insulin, the blood-sugar-lowering effect usually lasts from 24 to 28 hours, and the greatest effect occurs about 8 to 12 hours after the injection.

Lente insulin and NPH insulin are similar in action. Both have been found to suit the needs of a large percentage of patients.

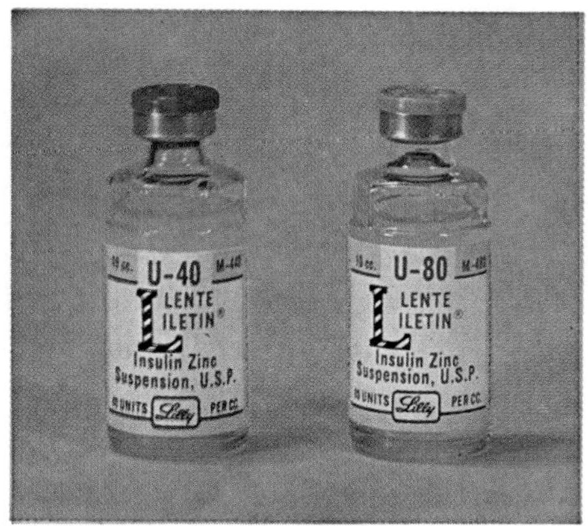

PLATE 5. Lente insulin for intermediate effect. (Eli Lilly & Co.)

Other Lente Insulin Preparations

There are two additional lente insulin preparations, one named semilente insulin and the other ultralente insulin. These are seldom used alone. When there is indication for their use, they are added to the lente insulin in the form of a mixture. The preparation of the mixtures of lente insulin with either semilente or ultralente insulin is discussed and illustrated on page 127, Insulin Mixtures.

Semilente Insulin

Semilente insulin is a cloudy, milky appearing solution contained in a round bottle with 6-sided shoulders (Hexanek). A large "S" in black print is superimposed on the colored printing of the label. The action of semilente insulin is rapid and lasts from 12 to 16 hours. Semilente insulin is particularly useful in speeding the action of lente insulin when the two are combined. The mixtures of these two preparations is indicated when better "after meal" control of the diabetes is needed.

Ultralente

Ultralente insulin is a cloudy, milky-appearing solution contained in a round bottle with 6-sided shoulders (Hexanek). A large "U" in black print is superimposed on the colored printing of the label. The action of ultralente insulin is slower and longer than that of lente insulin and closely resembles the action of protamine zinc insulin. Its greatest advantage concerns its use in the form of a mixture with lente insulin for patients who require further diabetic control in the early morning fasting condition.

TABLE 13. THE VARIOUS KINDS OF INSULIN PREPARATIONS, SHAPE OF THE BOTTLE, COLOR OF THE SOLUTION, DURATION OF THE BLOOD-SUGAR-LOWERING EFFECT AND THE TIME OF GREATEST EFFECT

KINDS OF INSULIN PREPARATIONS	SHAPE OF THE BOTTLE	COLOR OF THE SOLUTION	DURATION OF THE BLOOD-SUGAR-LOWERING EFFECT	TIME OF GREATEST EFFECT
Insulin (unmodified or regular)	Round	Clear	5 to 7 hours	2 to 3 hours
Protamine Zinc Insulin	Round	Cloudy, milky	36 to 48 hours	14 to 20 hours
Globin Insulin	Round	Clear, amber	Up to 24 hours	8 to 16 hours
NPH Insulin	Square	Cloudy, milky	24 to 28 hours	8 to 12 hours
Lente Insulin	Round with 6-sided shoulder	Cloudy, milky	24 to 28 hours	8 to 12 hours

DIVISION OF FOOD IN THE DIET WITH INSULIN THERAPY

The division of food in the diet needs careful consideration, especially when insulin therapy is required. The food intake should be arranged in meals so as to provide a fairly equal distribution of carbohydrate, protein and fat throughout the day. In addition to the morning, noon and night meals, intermediate feedings should be planned with regard to the insulin preparation that is prescribed. The division of daily food spaced more evenly over a longer period of time facilitates its usefulness and effectiveness. Furthermore, the possibility of insulin reaction is minimized (p. 136).

Usually, it is recommended that the meals be spaced from about 5 to 6 hours apart. The number of intermediate feedings and the times at which they are to be taken are dependent not only upon the kind of insulin used but also upon the needs of the individual patient. The particular requirements of the patient are always determined by the physician. The following discussion concerning meals and intermediate feedings, therefore, contains over-all general statements.

Rapid-Acting Insulin:

Insulin (Unmodified Insulin or Regular Insulin)

When only unmodified insulin is used, the patient should have 3 meals during the day, spaced from 5 to 6 hours apart. The division of the total food for the day is suggested in THE MEAL PLAN, page 65.

Long-Acting Insulin:

Protamine Zinc Insulin

When protamine zinc insulin is used, in addition to the 3 meals, spaced from 5 to 6 hours apart, there should be included a luncheon or feeding before bedtime. Often a small midmorning and/or midafternoon feeding is recommended as well. These feedings, especially the one before bedtime, are most important in preventing insulin reactions (p. 136).

While the midmorning and midafternoon feedings can be made up of simply a serving of fruit or a glass of milk, the feeding before bedtime should contain foods that will be absorbed over a longer period of time. These feedings can consist of milk and bread, crackers or cereal; or tea or coffee and cheese with bread or crackers; or fruit, cereal and milk or similar combinations of carbohydrate, protein and fat.

The Intermediate-Acting Insulins: Globin Insulin, NPH Insulin and Lente Insulin

When intermediate-acting insulins are used, in addition to the 3 meals, spaced from 5 to 6 hours apart, there should be included a luncheon or feeding in the midafternoon. Often, when indicated, a small midmorning and/or before bedtime feeding is recommended as well. These feedings, especially the midafternoon feeding, are important in the prevention of insulin reactions (p. 136).

While the midmorning and bedtime feedings can consist of a serving of fruit or a glass of milk, the midafternoon feeding should be somewhat larger. Milk and bread, crackers or cereal; or tea or coffee and cheese with bread or crackers; or fruit, cereal, and milk; or similar combinations of foods are usually recommended.

MEASUREMENT OF INSULIN

Strengths of Insulin Preparations

The strength of an insulin preparation is determined by the concentration which is measured in units. An insulin unit is a standard amount of insulin which has been determined by scientists and is the measurement used throughout the world. The strength of an insulin preparation is designated according to the number of units of insulin contained in each cubic centimeter.

Insulin preparations are available in two strengths. One of these, called U-40, has 40 units of insulin in each cubic centimeter; and the other, called U-80, has 80 units in each cubic centimeter. Every bottle of insulin contains 10 cubic centimeters. Therefore, a bottle of U-40 insulin has a total of 400 units (40 times 10), and a bottle of U-80 insulin has a total of 800 units (80 times 10). In other words, U-80 has twice the strength of U-40 or twice as many insulin units in each bottle.

There are two ways of recognizing the strengths of insulin preparations: one, by the label on the bottle which states the number of units of insulin in each cubic centimeter of solution, and the other by the colors used to identify the different strengths. U-40 insulin has a red label or red printing on the label and a red stopper. U-80 has a green label or green printing on the label and a green stopper. These colors are used universally to identify the strengths of insulins.

A Cubic Centimeter

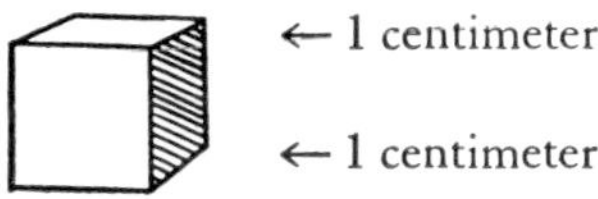

The volume of a cube which is 1 centimeter high, 1 centimeter wide and 1 centimeter deep is a cubic centimeter (cc.).

A centimeter is 1/100 of a meter.

A meter is about 3 inches longer than a yard.

THE SYRINGES FOR INSULIN

The physician always prescribes the type, the strength and the number of units of insulin to be used. It is then the responsibility of the patient to measure accurately the prescribed amount of insulin for each injection.

Of the many syringes manufactured, the one most commonly used is the "Official Insulin Syringe" recommended by the American Diabetes Association. It is most important that the patient know the meanings of the markings and the figures on the syringe he uses, to be certain that the amount of insulin measured corresponds to the amount prescribed. *When in doubt concerning the measurement of insulin, the physician should be consulted.*

Official Insulin Syringes

The Official Insulin Syringes that measure 1.0-cc. of insulin are manufactured in two types: a short type and a long type. The markings on the long-type syringes are farther apart, which allows them to be read with greater ease and with less margin of error. The long-type syringe is preferable, especially for those patients who have difficulties in vision.

The illustrations that follow show the long-type (Figs. 9 and 10) and the short-type (Figs. 11 and 12) Official Insulin Syringes and also indicate how insulin is measured.

Official Insulin Syringes—1-cc. Long Type*

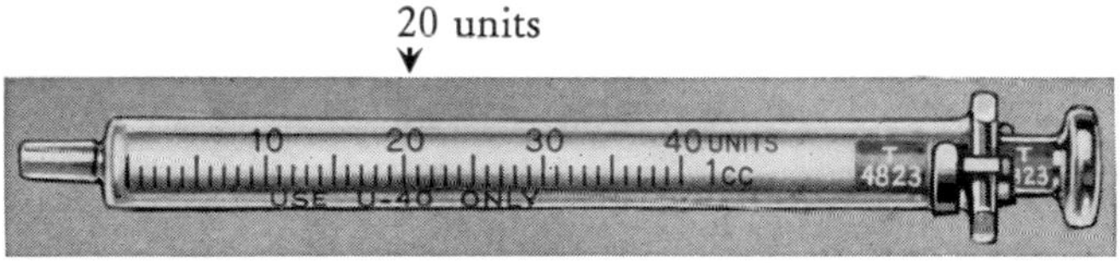

20 units

Fig. 9. Official Insulin Syringe—1-cc. long type for U-40 insulin,* showing how 20 units of insulin can be measured (single red scale).

20 units

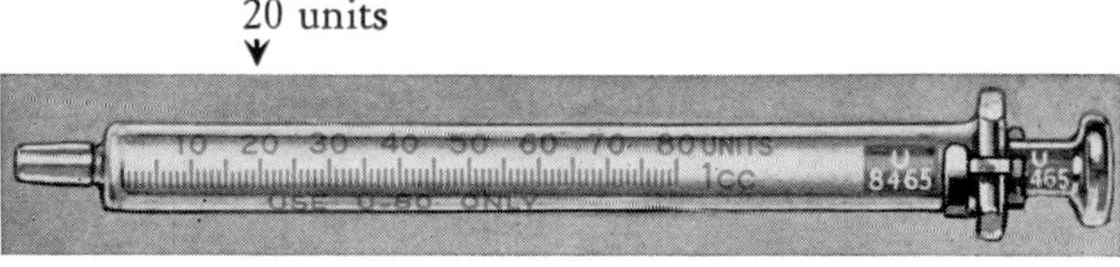

Fig. 10. Official Insulin Syringe—1-cc. long type for U-80 insulin,* showing how 20 units of insulin can be measured (single green scale).

* Becton, Dickinson & Co.

Official Insulin Syringes—1-cc. Short Type*

20 units

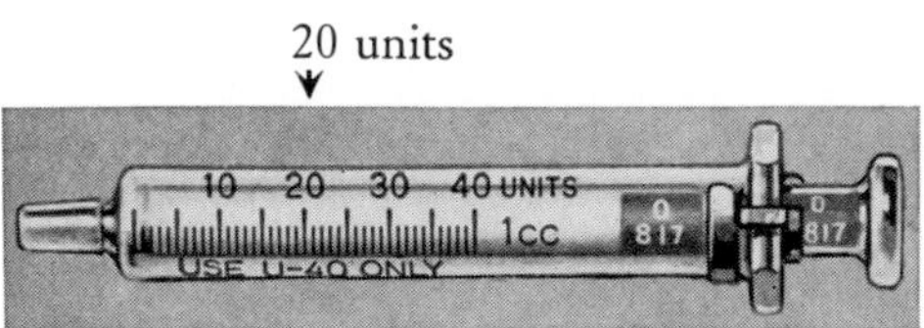

Fig. 11. Official Insulin Syringe—1-cc. short type for U-40 insulin,* showing how 20 units of insulin can be measured (single red scale).

20 units

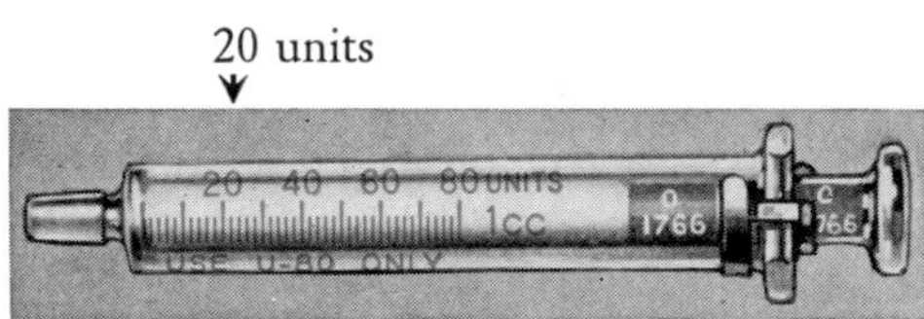

Fig. 12. Official Insulin Syringe—1-cc. short type for U-80 insulin,* showing how 20 units of insulin can be measured (single green scale).

When more than 1 cc. of U-80 insulin is required, the Official Insulin Syringe containing 2 cc. should be used. This long-type syringe is marked in a single scale (Fig. 13).

Official Insulin Syringe—2-cc.

120 units

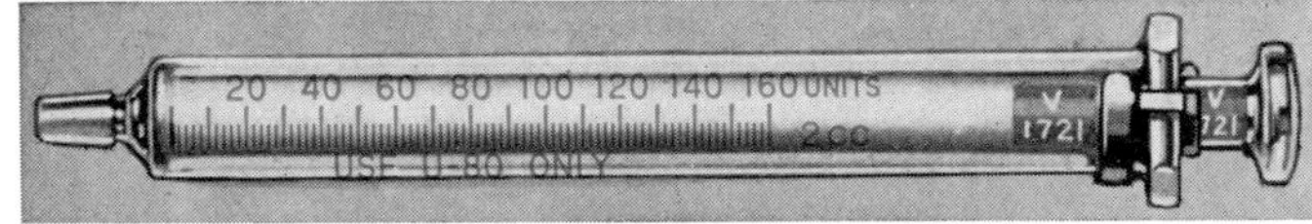

Fig. 13. Official Insulin Syringe 2-cc. for U-80 insulin, showing how 120 units of insulin can be measured (single green scale).*

* Becton, Dickinson & Co.

OTHER SYRINGES FOR INSULIN

There are other syringes which have marked on them one or more scales of figures to measure either the amount or the number of units of insulin. It is most important for the patient to know the meanings of the markings and the figures on the syringe he uses to be sure that the insulin measured corresponds to the amount prescribed. When in doubt concerning the measurement of insulin, the physician should be consulted to make certain that the insulin is measured correctly.

THE AUTOMATIC INJECTOR

There are available automatic injectors which may be preferred by the patient and recommended by the physician. The patient should be as thoroughly familiar with the correct technique when using an automatic injector as with other methods of insulin administration.

The syringe is filled with the correct amount of insulin, following the procedures on page 105. Then the needle is inserted into the skin automatically, according to the instructions. The plunger is pushed down to inject the insulin.

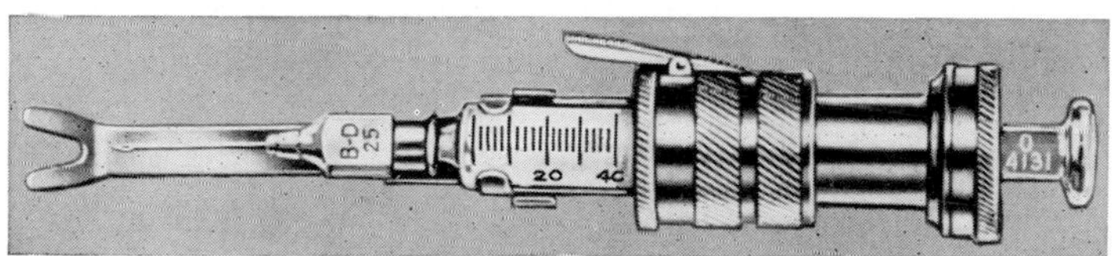

Fig. 14. Diagram of the Busher automatic injector. (Becton, Dickinson & Co.)

SPECIAL EQUIPMENT

There is special equipment which includes articles designed to aid in solving or decreasing problems resulting either from impaired vision or blindness. Of those available three are described, namely "C-Better Magnifier," "Insulin Syringe With Tru-Set Control" and "Insulin Needle Guide."

The C-Better Magnifier* is a small, plastic magnifier which is snapped on to the barrel of the syringe. The markings on the syringe are thereby magnified to almost twice the size so that the measurement of insulin can be more precise.

The Insulin Syringe With Tru-Set Control† has a device which can be set for the patient without sight so that he can be certain of the correct measurement of insulin.

The Insulin Needle Guide† is designed to assist the patient without sight in locating the center of the rubber stopper on the insulin vial.

* C-Better Magnifier can be obtained from Miss Marion Tschischeck, R.N., Jensen Beach, Florida.

† This equipment can be obtained from The American Foundation for the Blind, Inc., 15 West 16th Street, New York, New York.

THE HYPODERMIC NEEDLE FOR THE INJECTION OF INSULIN

A number of suitable brands of hypodermic needles are available for the injection of insulin. These are made of stainless steel which does not rust and requires a minimum of care. The needles that are recommended and commonly used are $\frac{3}{8}$, $\frac{1}{2}$ or $\frac{5}{8}$ inches in length, and they can be either 25 or 26 gauge.

Wires are provided that can be used for cleaning the bores and also may be inserted in the needles when they are not in use. The point of the needle must always be protected (see Injection of Insulin, p. 105) and when the needle has a dull or rough point it should be discarded. It is advisable to keep a reserve supply so that the insulin injection is not delayed through any mishap to the only needle.

INJECTION KITS

There are kits which contain the equipment necessary for the insulin injection. These have been designed to hold the insulin bottle, the syringe, the needles, as well as cotton and alcohol needed for sterilization. These kits are especially convenient when traveling or for use at home when facilities are limited.

DISPOSABLE INSULIN EQUIPMENT

There are available disposable needles and syringes with needles attached,* which are ready for a single use. This equipment is handy when home facilities are limited or when traveling.

The patient should use care in discarding hypodermic equipment to make certain there is no risk of its use for other purposes. It is recommended that this material be totally destroyed by incineration or other means.

* Becton, Dickinson & Co.

PROCEDURE FOR INJECTION OF INSULIN

The correct method of the injection of insulin should be understood. At first, this procedure requires a great deal of care, since there are many details that must be known. However, once familiar with the steps for injection of insulin, the procedure is done with ease and becomes a matter of routine.

1. *A tray set up with the necessary equipment* should be kept in a handy place ready for use. The tray and the various articles should be clean at all times. The articles necessary for the injection of insulin are: bottle of insulin, bottle of alcohol, dish to hold alcohol, clean absorbent cotton in a covered container and the needle and the syringe in their box (Fig. 15).

2. *Cleanliness* is a rule of prime importance from the first to the last step of the procedure for the injection of insulin and must not be overlooked. In preparation, the hands should be washed carefully with mild soap and warm water and should be dried with a clean towel (Fig. 16).

3. *Alcohol* is used to sterilize* the necessary articles for the injection of insulin. Articles requiring sterilization are: the top of the bottle of insulin,† the needle and the syringe. The skin where the injection is to be made must also be sterilized with absorbent cotton dipped in alcohol. The alcohol is poured into a clean dish for this purpose (Fig. 17).

4. *It is necessary that the contents of the bottles of protamine zinc insulin, NPH insulin and lente insulin be well mixed before using.* This is done by rolling the bottle between the palms of the hands, but not shaking it, since by so doing the insulin would foam. This procedure is not necessary for other kinds of insulin (Fig. 18).

5. *The whole top of the bottle of insulin is sterilized* by dipping it in the dish of alcohol or wiping it with a small piece of cotton soaked with alcohol. This must always be done before inserting the needle in the stopper. The rubber stopper in the insulin bottle keeps the insulin sterile and never should be removed (Fig. 19).

6. *It is well to keep a wire in the needle* to prevent it from becoming plugged. The wire should always be removed from the needle before it is sterilized (Fig. 20).

7. *The needle* should be placed carefully in the alcohol* so that the point will not be blunted by hitting the dish. Dull needles should not be used, since they may injure the skin. The needle should remain in the alcohol until it is placed on the syringe (Fig. 21).

8. *The syringe for the injection of insulin* consists of a barrel, which is like a cylinder or a tube, and a

* Medicated "rubbing" 70 per cent ethyl alcohol or isopropyl alcohol may be used. Denatured alcohol should not be used.

† Each insulin bottle has a protective aluminum seal. The directions for removing this seal are found on the instruction pamphlet contained in the insulin package.

* 25-gauge or 26-gauge, 3/8, 1/2 or 5/8 inch needle, preferably stainless steel.

plunger, which is a glass rod that fits into the barrel (Fig. 22).

9. *The syringe is put together* for the injection of insulin by inserting the plunger in the barrel. The plunger (glass rod) should fit snugly into the barrel of the syringe, so that there is no leakage of insulin (Fig. 23).

10. *The syringe is then sterilized with alcohol.* This is accomplished by placing the end of the syringe in the dish of alcohol and drawing up the plunger to fill the syringe with the alcohol, and then pushing the plunger down to empty it. This should be repeated 3 or 4 times (Fig. 24).

11. *The needle is placed firmly on the syringe* by twisting it to make it secure. The needle is held by the hub to keep the point sterile since it should not be touched by the hands or come in contact with any object (Fig. 25).

12. *The syringe and the needle must be completely emptied of all alcohol.* This is done by pulling the plunger up and down several times until the syringe and the needle are thoroughly dry (Fig. 26).

13. *It is necessary to replace with the same amount of air the amount of insulin to be withdrawn from the bottle.* The syringe is filled with air by drawing the plunger as far as the figure that measures the amount of insulin that has been prescribed (Fig. 27).

14. *The air in the syringe is forced into the bottle* by inserting the needle through the center of the stopper of the insulin bottle. The syringe should be held near the needle and in a straight line with the insulin bottle so that the needle will not become bent as it is pushed through the stopper (Fig. 28).

15. *Air is forced into the bottle* by pushing the plunger of the syringe as far as it will go. When the air is not forced into the insulin bottle to replace the insulin to be withdrawn from it, a vacuum is created in the bottle. A vacuum in the bottle makes it difficult to pull the plunger when measuring insulin because the plunger is sucked back as it is pulled (Fig. 29).

16. *The syringe is filled with insulin* by drawing the plunger as far as the figure that measures the amount of insulin prescribed. One hand is used to hold both the insulin bottle and syringe, allowing the other hand to be free to pull the plunger. The bottle of insulin is turned upside down so that the insulin is immediately over the stopper. To prevent bending the needle the insulin bottle and the syringe should be kept in a straight line. Care should be taken to have no air in the syringe, since it would take up space intended for insulin. If there is air in the syringe, it will appear as a bubble in the insulin. Whenever an air bubble appears the plunger should be pushed to force the air back into the bottle of insulin, and then pulled out again (Fig. 30).

17. *The needle is withdrawn from the bottle* (Fig. 31).

18. *The syringe, which is now filled with insulin, should be put down carefully* so that the needle on the syringe

does not touch the hand or any object. The cover of the syringe box with its cutouts is a good resting place for the syringe until the skin is sterilized for the injection of insulin (Fig. 32).

19. *The place of injection is changed with each injection of insulin.* First one leg or arm is used, and then the other. The abdomen may also be used. A place where an injection has been made should not be used again for months (Fig. 33).

20. *A small piece of absorbent cotton is dipped in the dish of alcohol* (Fig. 34).

21. *The skin is sterilized at the place of injection* by rubbing it gently with the cotton that has been soaked with alcohol (Fig. 35).

22. *The cotton may be placed back in the dish of alcohol or rested on the leg,* where it is ready to use again after the insulin has been injected (Fig. 36).

23. (A) *The left hand is used to pinch a large amount of flesh,* the center of which is to be used for the injection. With the flesh thus held firmly, the needle can be injected more easily (Fig. 37). (B) *The skin can be stretched* between the thumb and the first (index) finger when one is unable to pinch a large amount of flesh (Fig. 38).

24. *The needle is injected at a right angle (straight, not slanted) to the leg.* The syringe is held as one would hold a pencil, between the thumb and the index finger of the right hand, and the needle is pushed firmly for its entire length into the skin. Once the needle is injected into the skin it is not necessary to hold the flesh. With the left hand, pull the plunger of the syringe back gently, and if blood is drawn into the syringe, withdraw the needle and insert it elsewhere (Fig. 39).

25. *The right hand is used to hold the syringe steady while the left hand holds the syringe at the top, between the index and the middle fingers,* and the thumb pushes the plunger to inject the insulin (Fig. 40).

26. *The needle is withdrawn quickly with the right hand.* At the same time, the left hand, with the cotton that has been dipped in alcohol, presses the cotton firmly over the place of injection so that the needle will not pull the skin as it is withdrawn (Fig. 41).

27. *The skin is then sterilized* at the place of injection by rubbing it gently with the cotton that has been soaked with alcohol (Fig. 42).

28. *The needle is placed in the dish of alcohol* to keep it from becoming plugged. The needle should be placed carefully in the alcohol so that the point will not be blunted by hitting the dish (Fig. 43).

29. *The syringe is washed in alcohol* to prevent the plunger and the barrel from sticking. This is accomplished by placing the end of the syringe in the dish of alcohol and drawing up the plunger to fill the syringe with alcohol and then pushing the plunger down to empty it (Fig. 44).

30. *The syringe is placed carefully in its box* (Fig. 45).

31. *The wire is inserted in the needle* (Fig. 46).

32. *The needle is wrapped in cotton and placed in the box* (Fig. 47).

33. *The alcohol in the dish is poured back into the bottle,* since it can be used as long as it remains clear and does not become discolored. The neck of the alcohol bottle should be wide enough so that the alcohol may be poured back easily and not wasted (Fig. 48).

34. *It is well to boil the syringe in water every week.* In so doing, the bottom of the pan should be covered with a cloth to prevent the syringe from hitting against the pan and breaking; or the syringe may be placed in a strainer which has been set in water for this purpose. In certain parts of the country the syringe may become coated from boiling in the hard water. When only hard water is available these deposits can be prevented by the use of distilled water or by wrapping the syringe and the needle in cloth or gauze before boiling (Fig. 49).

35. *Insulin should not be subjected to extremes of temperature, and insulin bottles not in use should be stored in the refrigerator, but freezing should be avoided.* The bottle of insulin that is being used can be kept at ordinary room temperature (Fig. 50).

36. *The tray is left ready for the next injection.* The dish of cotton is covered, the bottle of alcohol closed, the dish for the alcohol turned upside down on the tray, the insulin bottle placed in the box, and the container for the syringe and needle covered (Fig. 51).

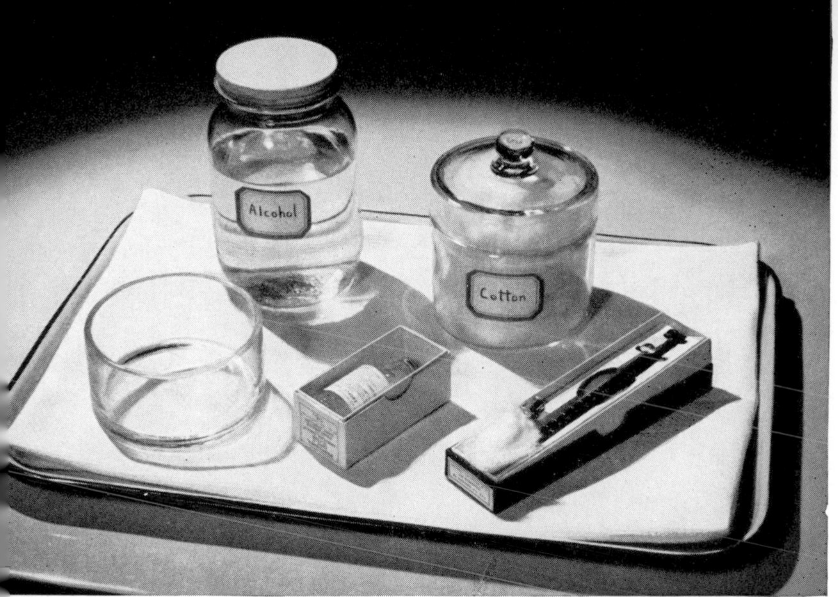

Fig. 15. *A tray set up with the necessary equipment* should be kept in a handy place ready for use. The tray and the various articles should be clean at all times. The articles necessary for the injection of insulin are: bottle of insulin, bottle of alcohol, dish to hold alcohol, clean absorbent cotton in a covered container and the needle and the syringe in their box.

Fig. 16. *Cleanliness* is a rule of prime importance from the first to the last step of the procedure for the injection of insulin and must not be overlooked. In preparation, the hands should be washed carefully with mild soap and warm water and should be dried with a clean towel.

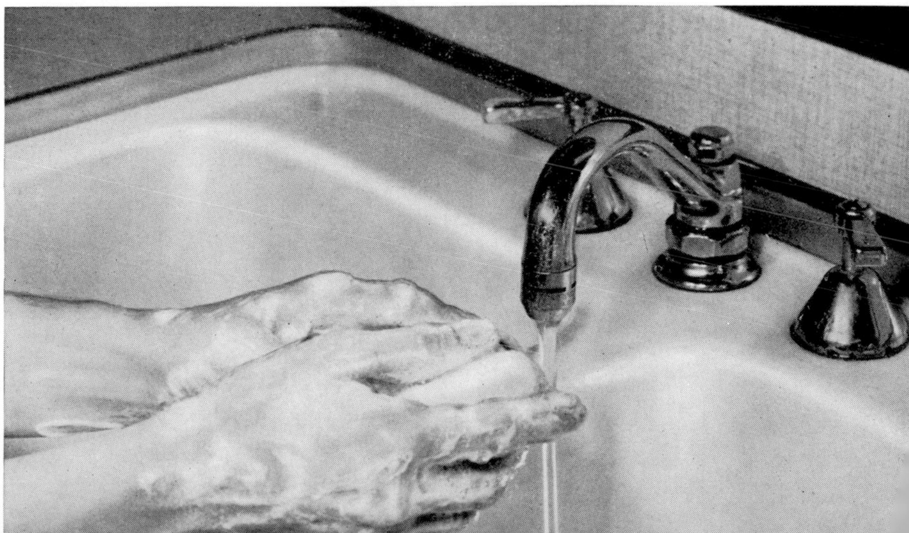

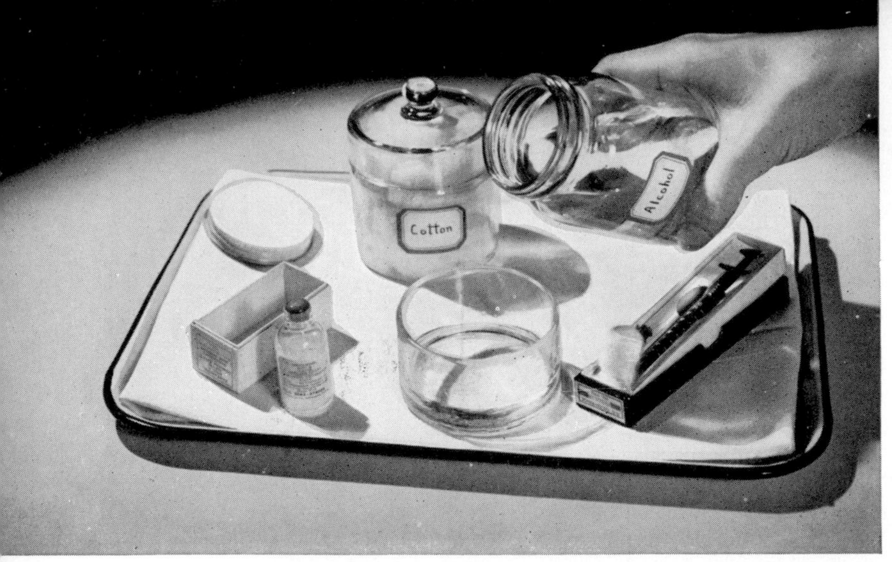

FIG. 17. *Alcohol is used to sterilize* the necessary articles for the injection of insulin. Articles requiring sterilization are: the top of the bottle of insulin, the needle and the syringe. The skin where the injection is to be made must also be sterilized with absorbent cotton dipped in alcohol. The alcohol is poured into a clean dish for this purpose.

FIG. 18. *It is necessary that the contents of the bottles of protamine zinc insulin, NPH insulin and lente insulin be well mixed before using*. This is done by rolling the bottle between the palms of the hands but not shaking it, since by so doing the insulin would foam. This procedure is not necessary for other kinds of insulin.

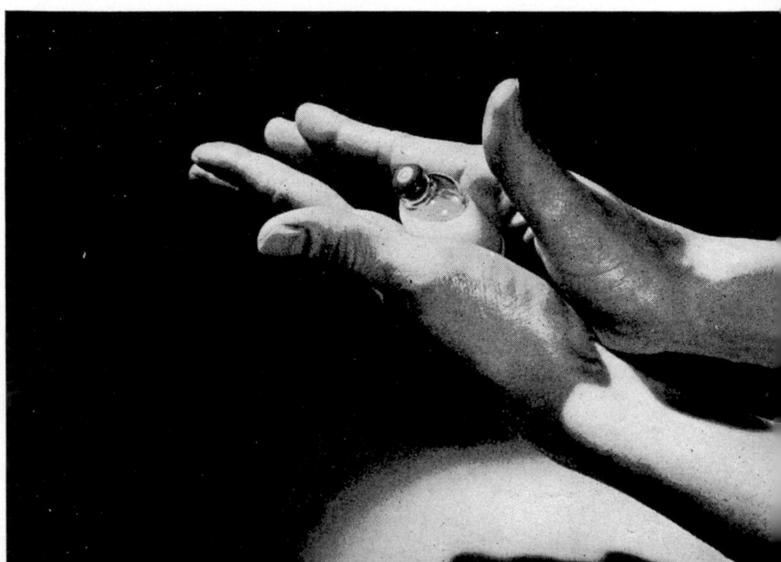

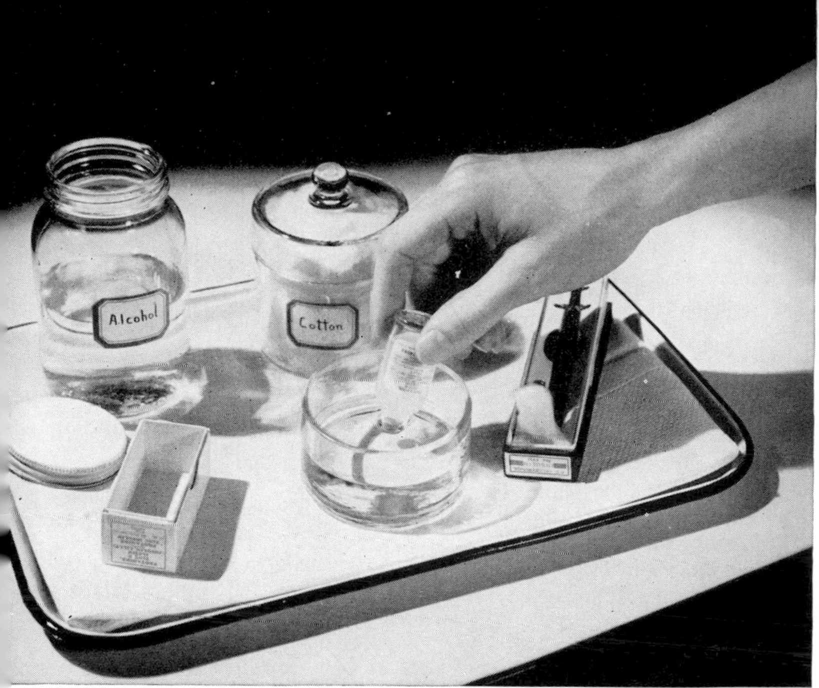

Fig. 19. *The whole top of the bottle of insulin is sterilized* by dipping it in the dish of alcohol. This must always be done before inserting the needle in the stopper. *The rubber stopper in the insulin bottle never should be removed because it keeps the insulin sterile.*

Fig. 20. *It is well to keep a wire in the needle* to prevent it from becoming plugged. The wire should always be removed from the needle before it is sterilized.

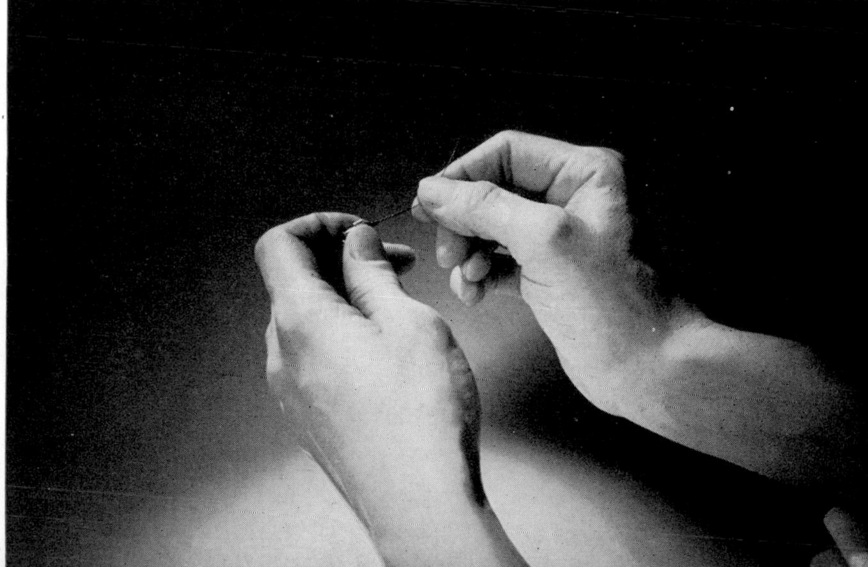

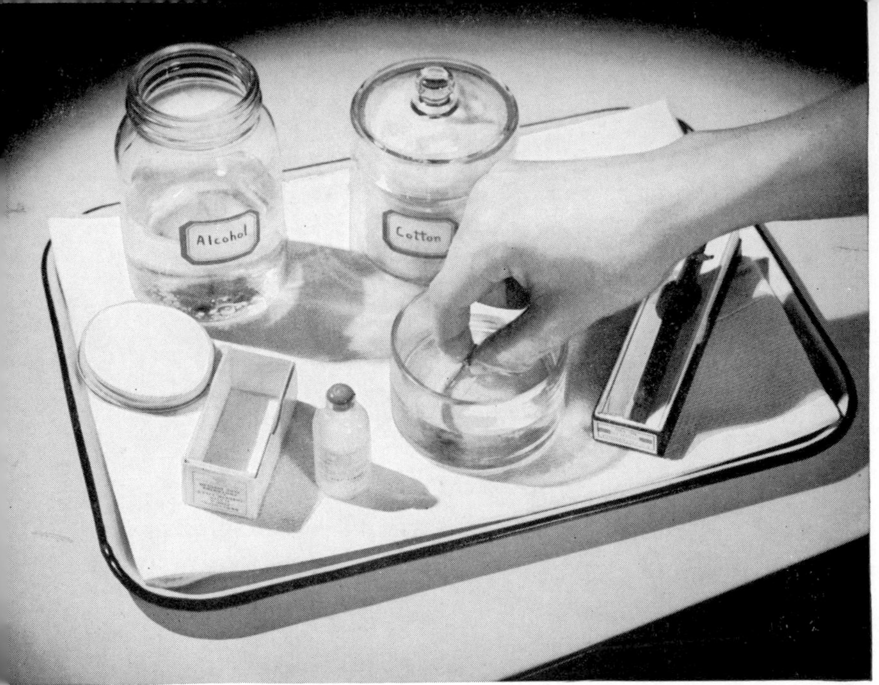

Fig. 21. *The needle should be placed carefully in the alcohol* so that the point will not be blunted by hitting the dish. Dull needles should not be used, since they may injure the skin. The needle should remain in the alcohol until ready to be placed on the syringe.

Fig. 22. *The syringe for the injection of insulin* consists of a barrel, which is like a cylinder or tube, and a plunger, which is a glass rod that fits into the barrel.

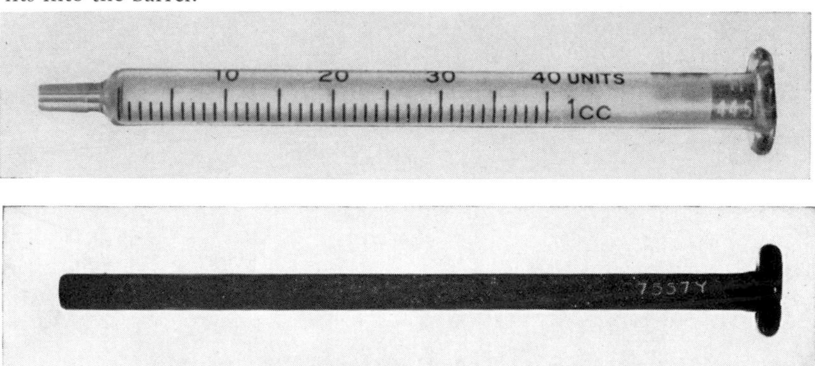

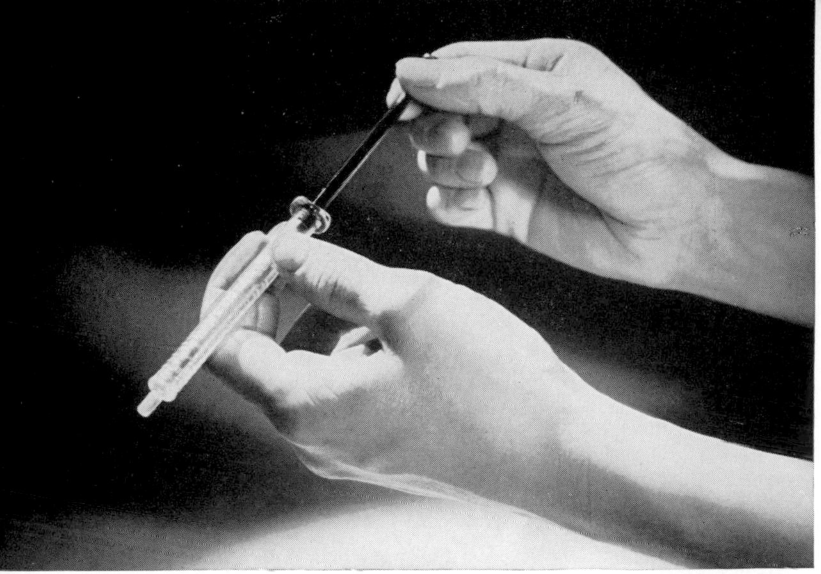

Fig. 23. *The syringe is put together* for the injection of insulin by inserting the plunger in the barrel. The plunger (glass rod) should fit snugly into the barrel of the syringe, so that there is no leakage of insulin.

Fig. 24. *The syringe is sterilized with alcohol.* This is accomplished by placing the end of the syringe in the dish of alcohol and drawing up the plunger to fill the syringe with the alcohol, and then pushing the plunger down to empty it. This should be repeated 3 or 4 times.

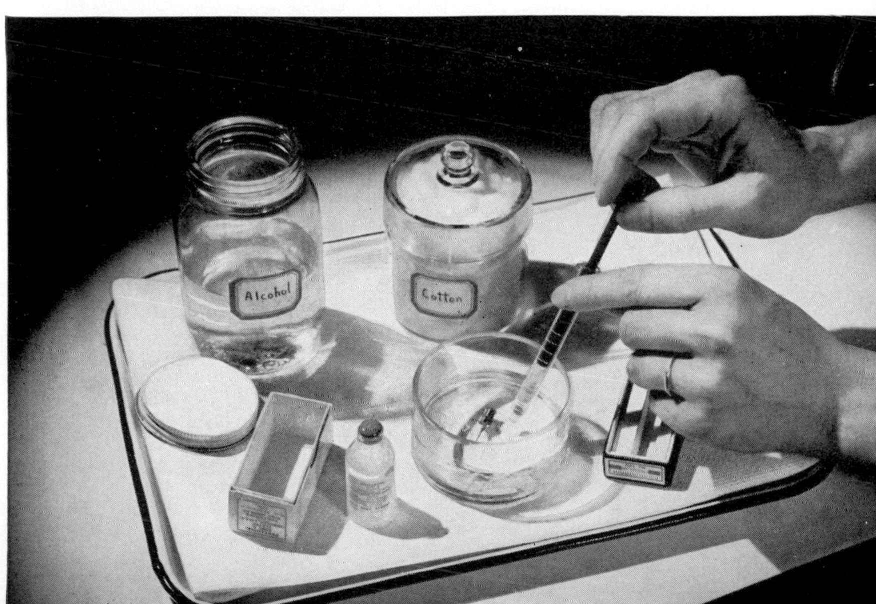

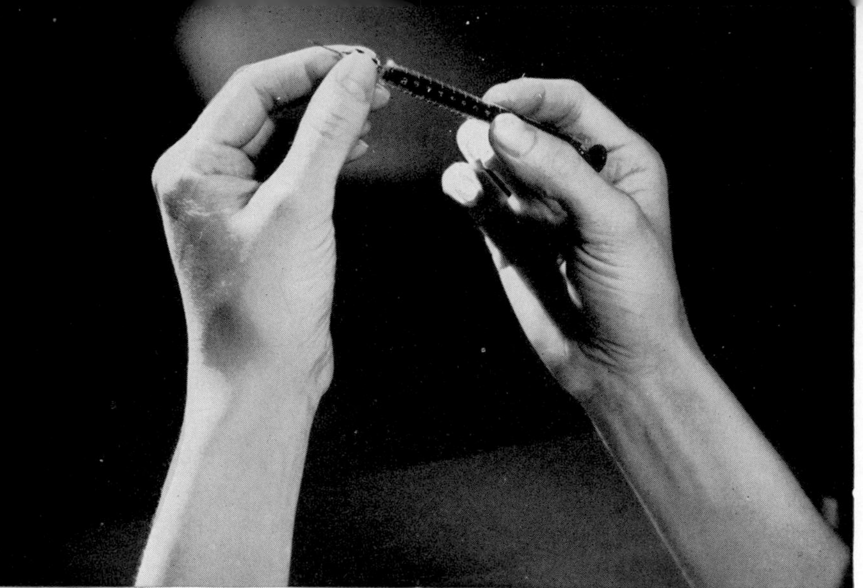

Fig. 25. *The needle is placed firmly on the syringe* by twisting it to make it secure. The needle is held by the hub to keep the point sterile since it should not be touched by the hands or come in contact with any object.

Fig. 26. *The syringe and the needle must be completely emptied of all alcohol.* This is done by pulling the plunger up and down several times until the syringe and the needle are thoroughly dry.

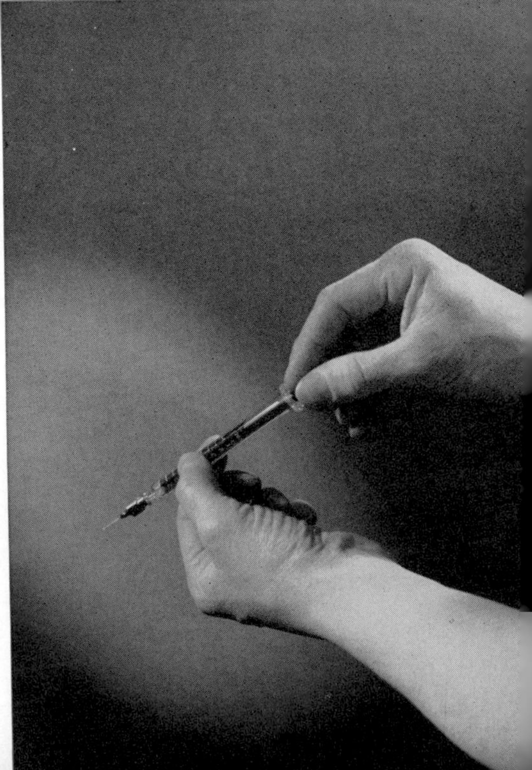

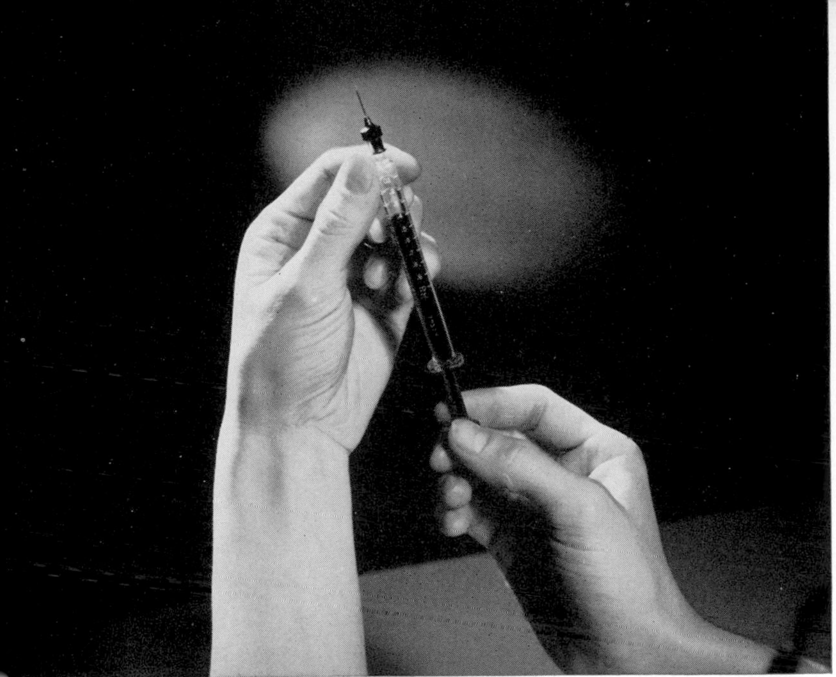

Fig. 27. *It is necessary to replace with the same amount of air the amount of insulin* to be withdrawn from the bottle. The syringe is filled with air by drawing the plunger as far as the figure that measures the amount of insulin that has been prescribed.

Fig. 28. *The air in the syringe is forced into the bottle* by inserting the needle through the center of the stopper of the insulin bottle. The syringe should be held near the needle and in a straight line with the insulin bottle so that the needle will not become bent as it is pushed through the stopper.

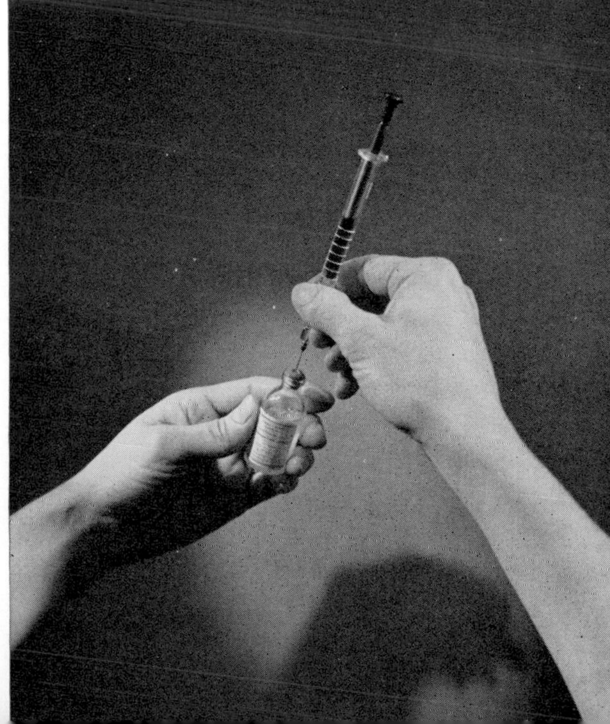

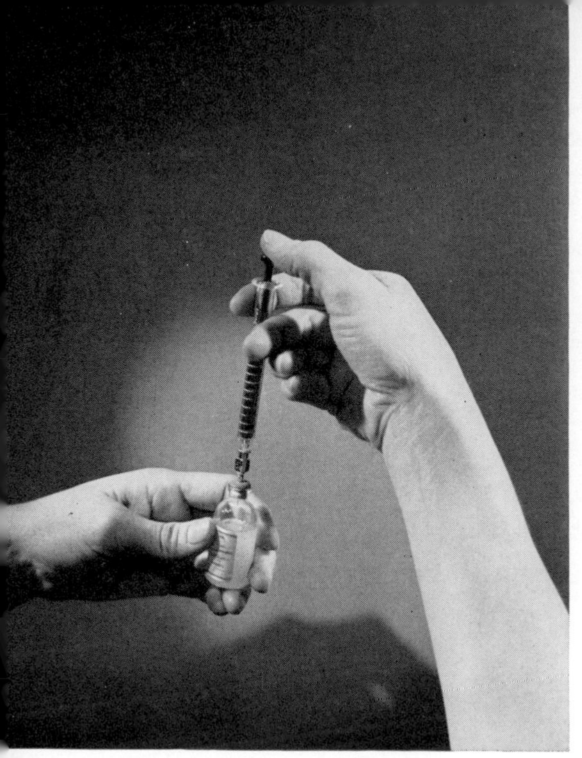

Fig 29. *Air is forced into the bottle* by pushing the plunger of the syringe as far as it will go. When air is not forced into the insulin bottle to replace the insulin to be withdrawn from it, a vacuum is created in the bottle. A vacuum in the bottle makes it difficult to pull the plunger when measuring insulin because the plunger is sucked back as it is pulled.

Fig. 30. *The syringe is filled with insulin* by drawing the plunger as far as the figure that measures the amount of insulin prescribed. One hand is used to hold both the insulin bottle and syringe, allowing the other hand to be free to pull the plunger. The bottle of insulin is turned upside down so that the insulin is immediately over the stopper. To prevent bending the needle the insulin bottle and the syringe should be kept in a straight line. Care should be taken to have no air in the syringe, since it would take up space intended for insulin. If there is air in the syringe, it will appear as a bubble in the insulin. Whenever an air bubble appears, the plunger should be pushed to force the air back into the bottle of insulin and then pulled out again.

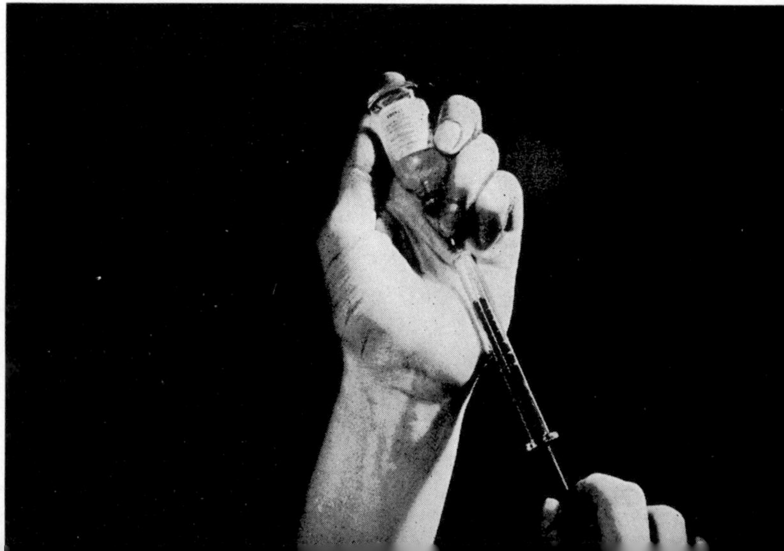

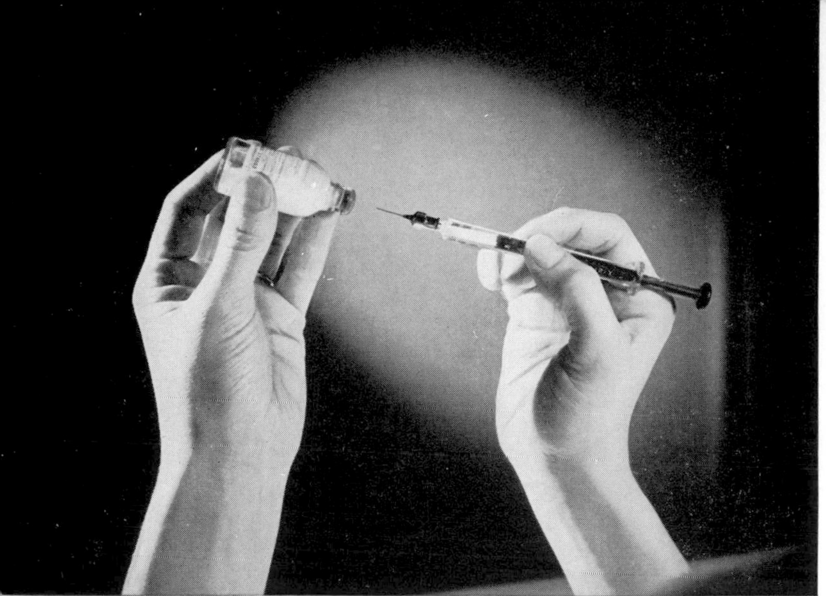

Fig. 31. *The needle is withdrawn from the bottle.*

Fig. 32. *The syringe, which is now filled with insulin, should be put down carefully* so that the needle on the syringe does not touch the hand or any object. The cover of the syringe box with its cutouts is a good resting place for the syringe until the skin is sterilized for the injection of insulin.

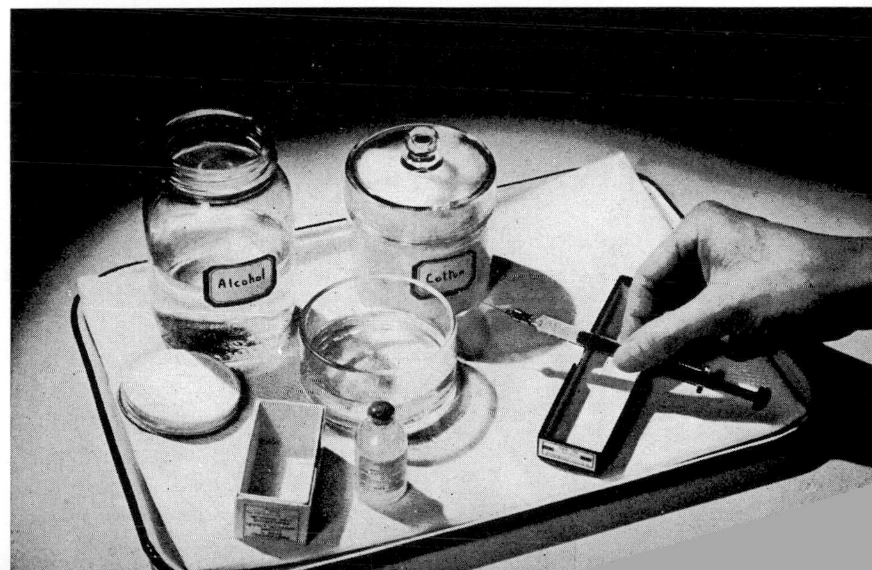

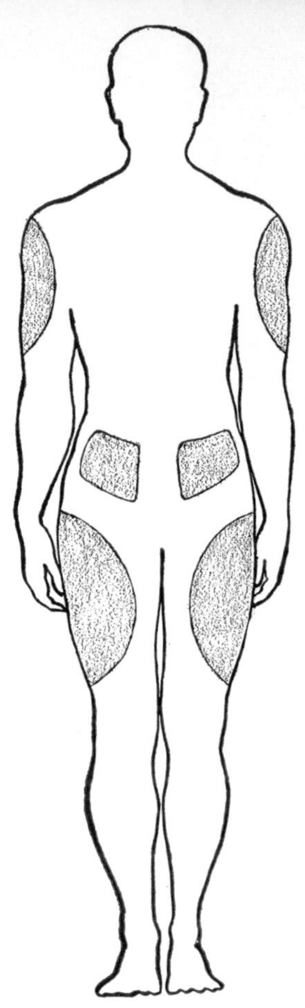

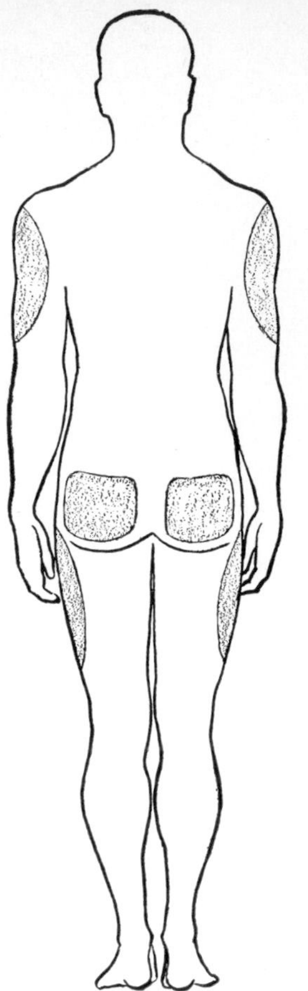

Fig. 33. *The place of injection is changed with each injection of insulin.* First one leg or arm is used, and then the other. The abdomen may be used also. A place where an injection has been made should not be used again for months.

Fig. 34. *A small piece of absorbent cotton is dipped in the dish of alcohol.*

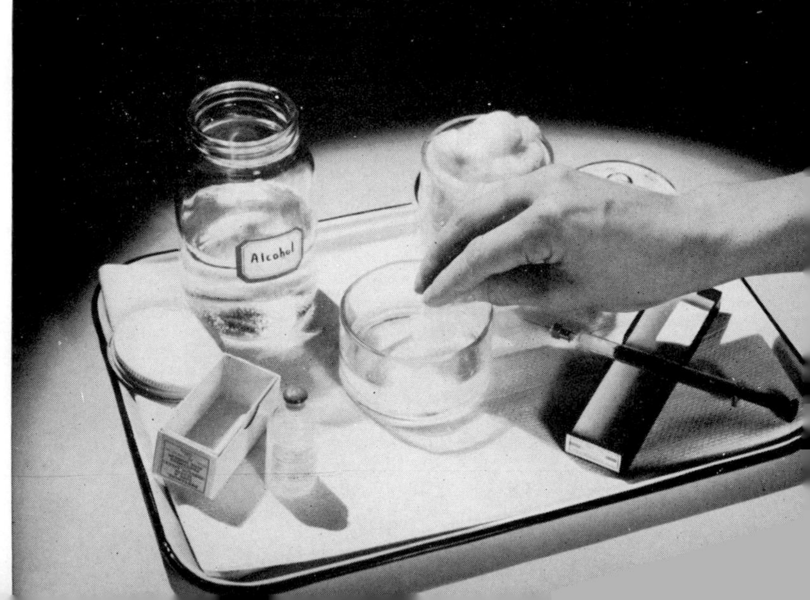

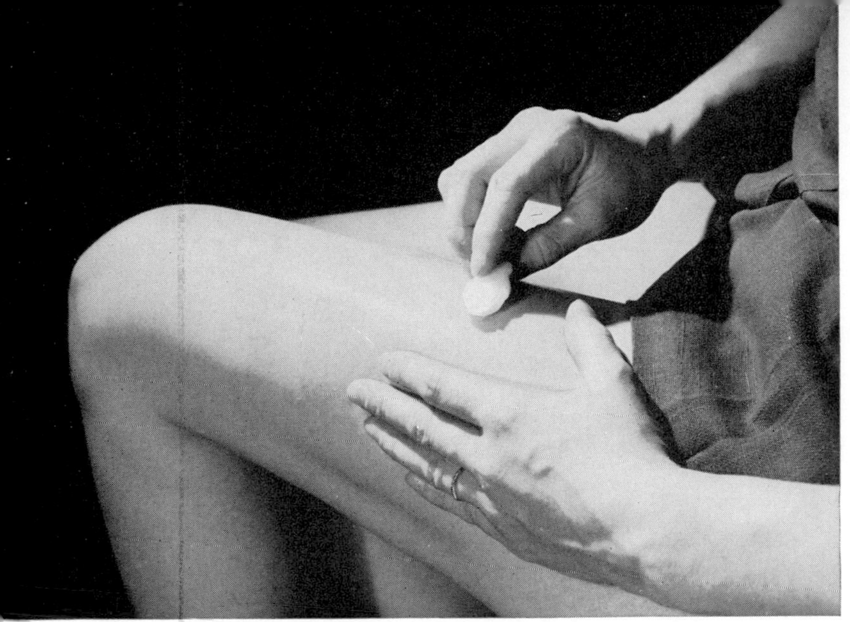

Fig. 35. *The skin is sterilized* at the place of injection by rubbing it gently with the cotton that has been soaked with alcohol.

Fig. 36. *The cotton may be placed back in the dish of alcohol or rested on the leg,* where it is ready to use again after the insulin has been injected.

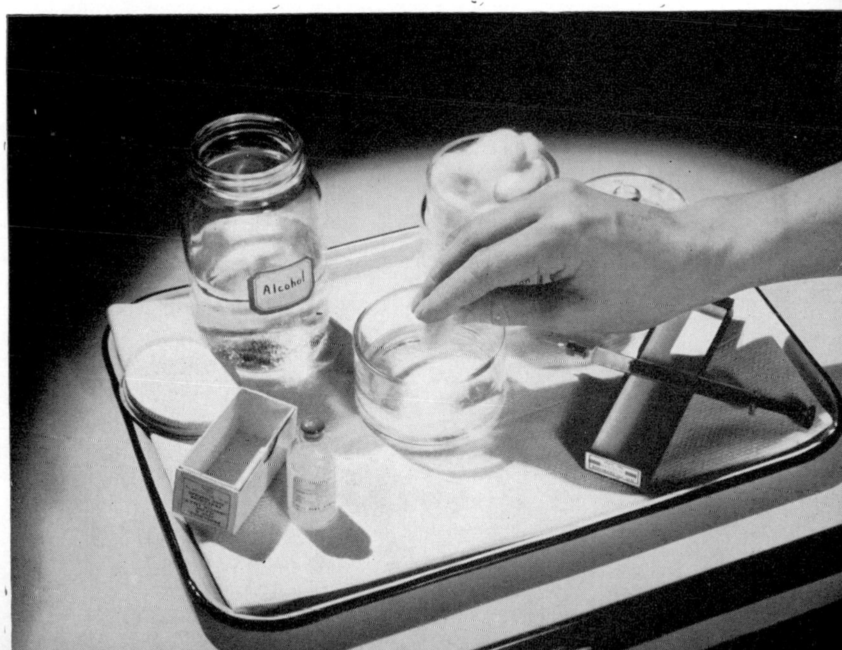

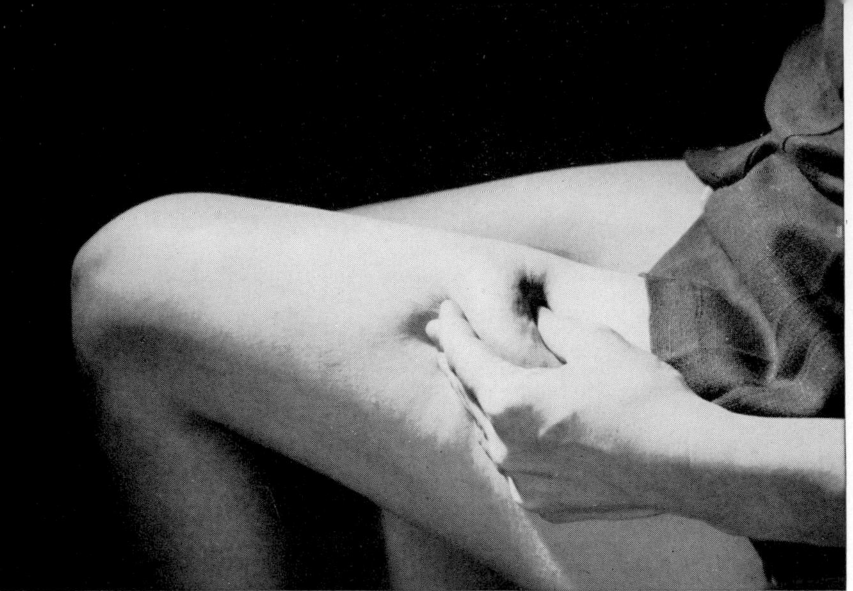

Fig. 37. *The left hand is used to pinch a large amount of flesh,* the center of which is to be used for the injection. With the flesh thus held firmly, the needle can be injected more easily.

Fig. 38. *The skin can be stretched* between the thumb and the first (index) finger when one is unable to pinch a large amount of flesh.

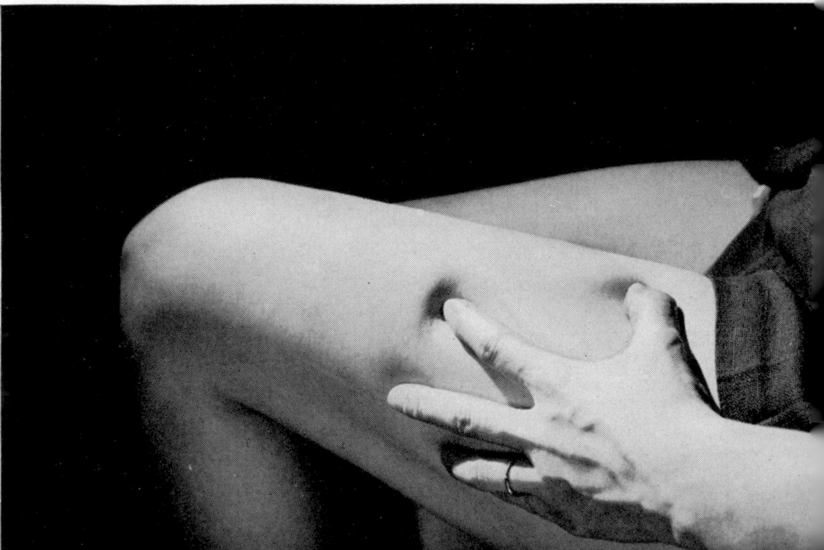

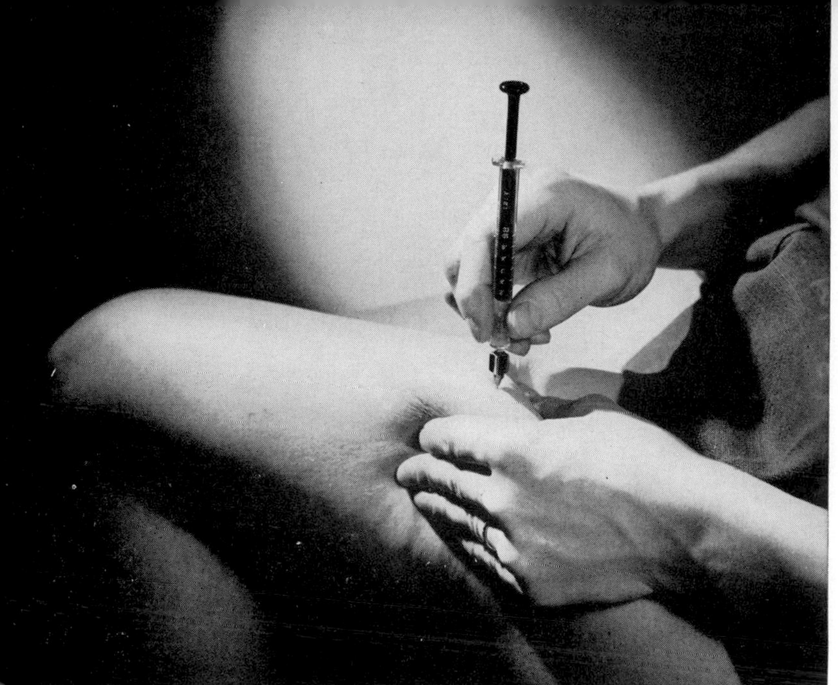

FIG. 39. *The needle is injected at a right angle (straight, not slanted) to the leg.* The syringe is held as one would hold a pencil, between the thumb and the index finger of the right hand, and the needle is pushed firmly for its entire length into the skin. Once the needle is injected into the skin it is not necessary to hold the flesh. With the left hand, pull the plunger of the syringe back gently, and if blood is drawn into the syringe, withdraw the needle and insert it elsewhere.

FIG. 40. *The right hand is used to hold the syringe steady while the left hand holds the syringe at the top, between the index and the middle fingers,* and the thumb pushes the plunger to inject the insulin.

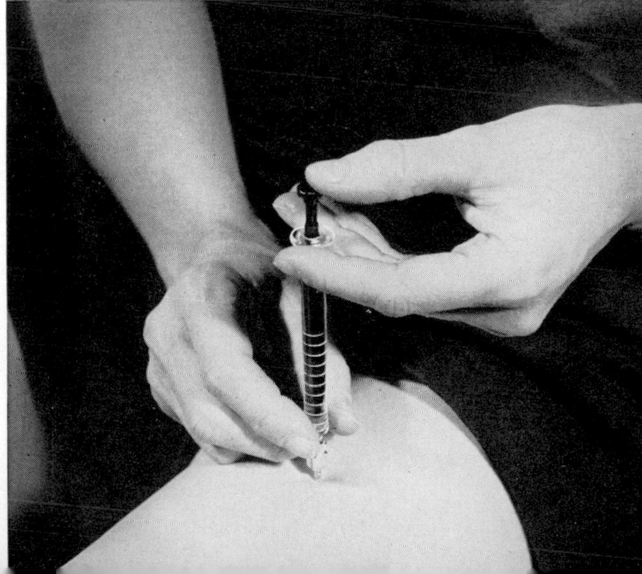

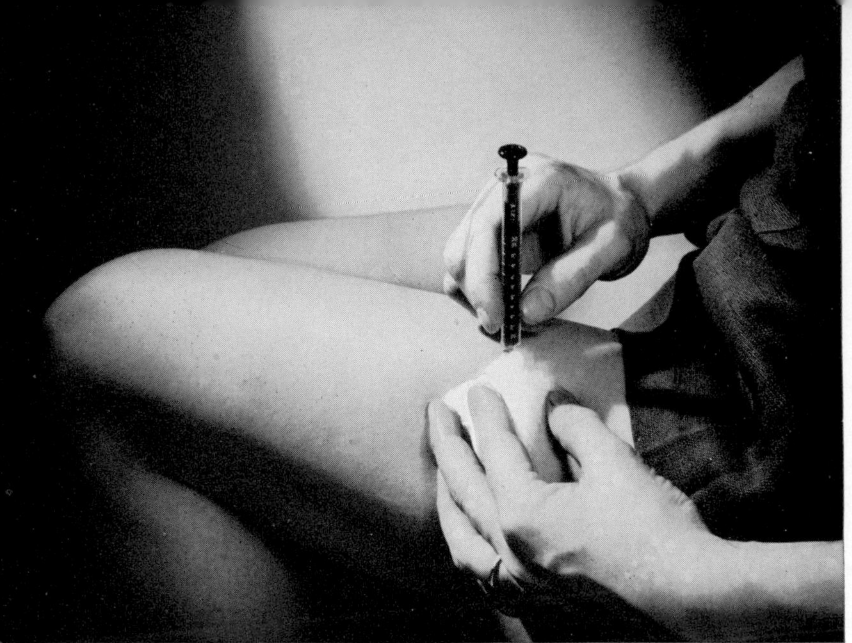

Fig. 41. *The needle is withdrawn quickly with the right hand.* At the same time, the left hand, with the cotton that has been dipped in alcohol, presses the cotton firmly over the place of injection so that the needle will not pull the skin as it is withdrawn.

Fig. 42. *The skin is sterilized* at the place of injection by rubbing it gently with the cotton that has been soaked with alcohol.

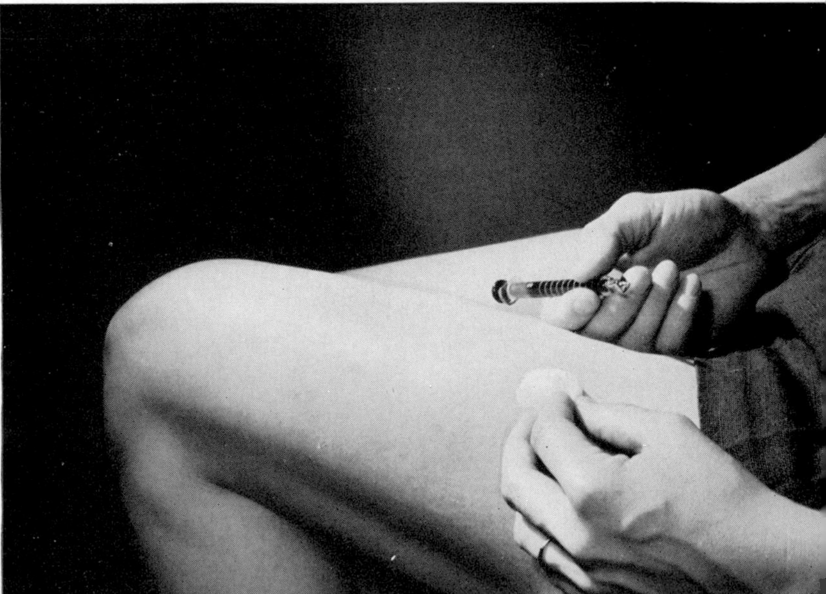

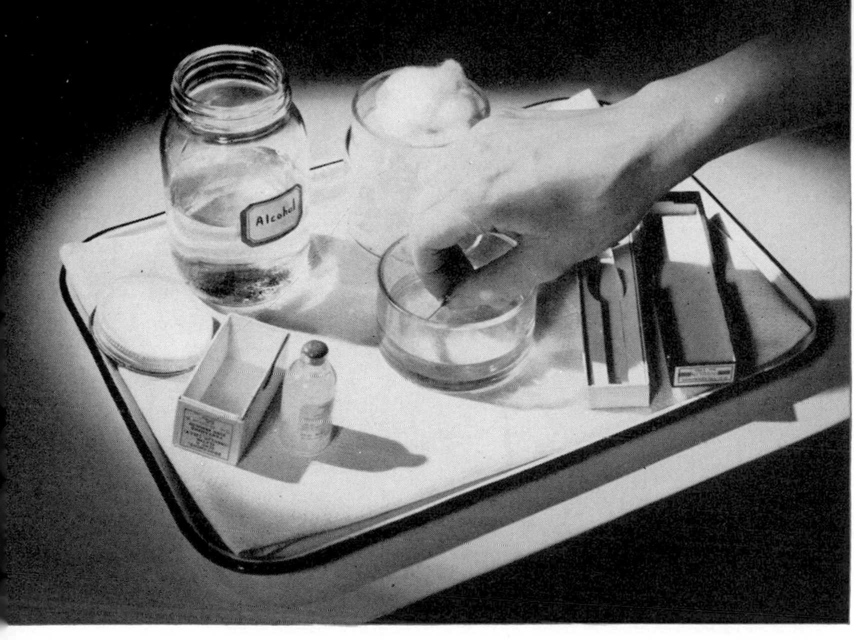

Fig. 43. *The needle is placed in the dish of alcohol* to keep it from becoming plugged. The needle should be placed carefully in the alcohol so that the point will not be blunted by hitting the dish.

Fig. 44. *The syringe is washed in alcohol* to prevent the plunger and the barrel from sticking. This is accomplished by placing the end of the syringe in the dish of alcohol and drawing up the plunger to fill the syringe with alcohol and then pushing the plunger down to empty it.

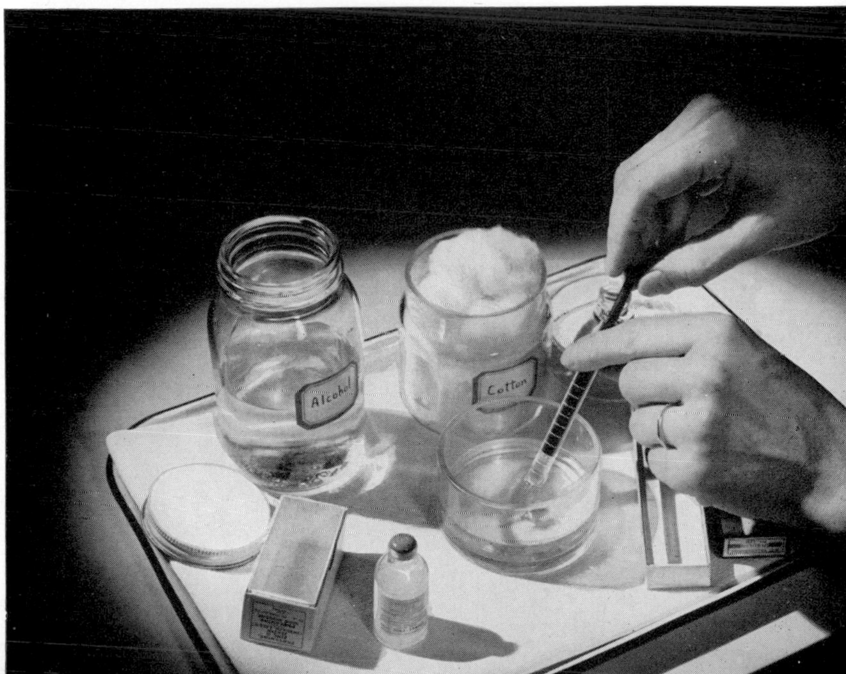

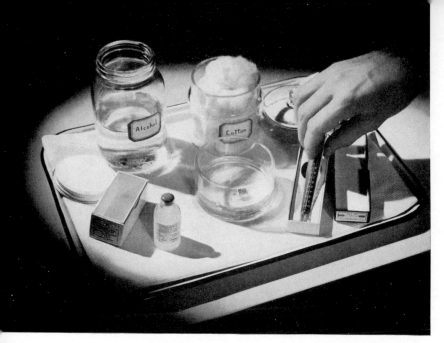

FIG. 45. *The syringe is placed carefully in its box.*

FIG. 46. *The wire is inserted in the needle.*

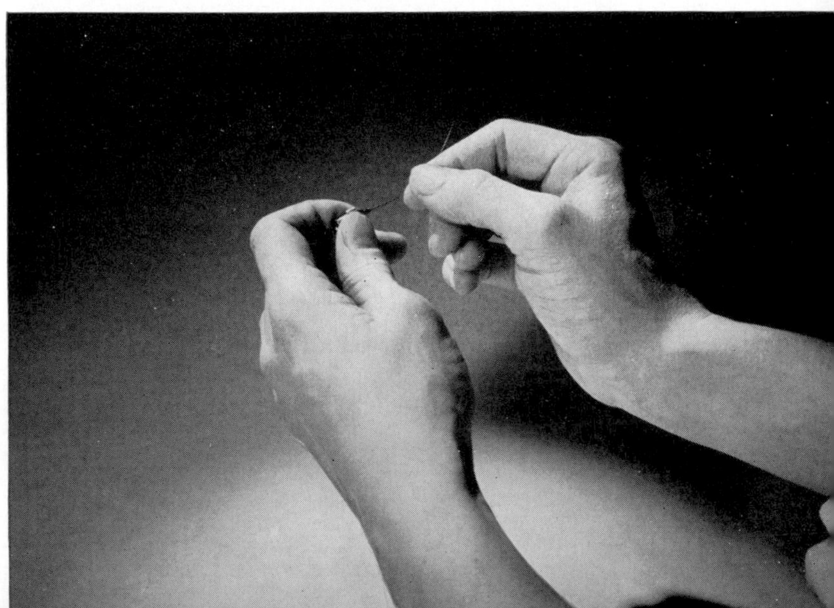

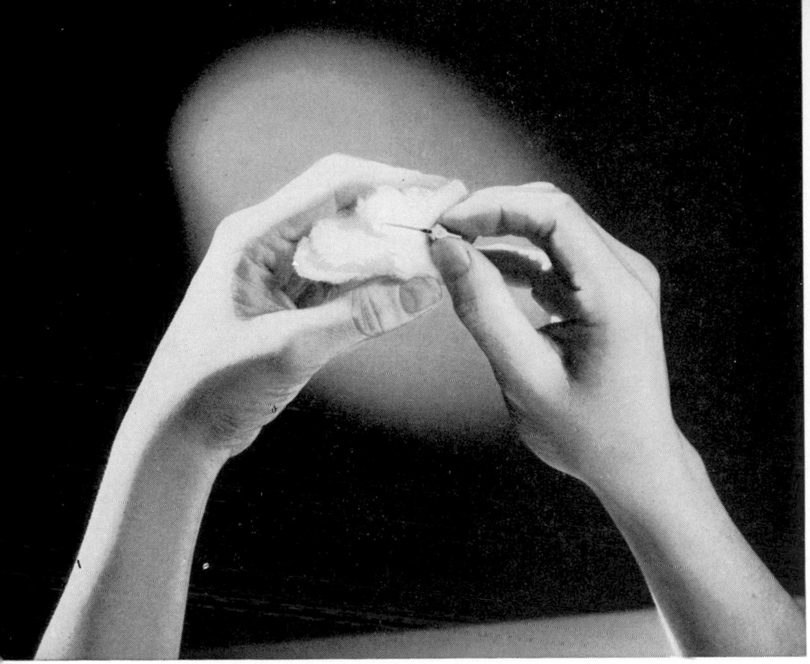

FIG. 47. *The needle is wrapped in cotton and placed in the box.*

FIG. 48. *The alcohol in the dish is poured back into the bottle,* since it can be used as long as it remains clear and does not become discolored. The neck of the alcohol bottle should be wide enough so that the alcohol may be poured back easily and not be wasted.

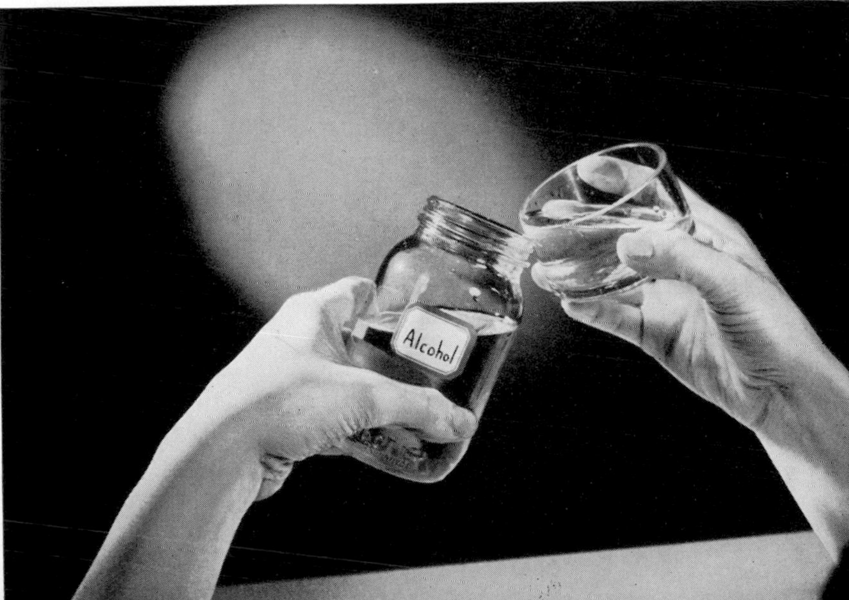

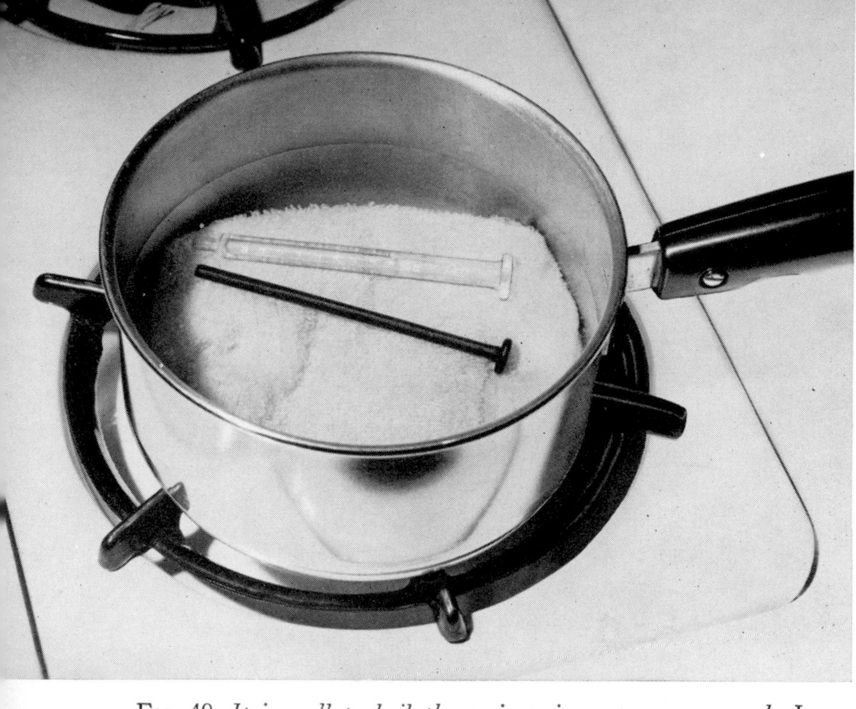

Fig. 49. *It is well to boil the syringe in water every week.* In so doing, the bottom of the pan should be covered with a cloth to prevent the syringe from hitting against the pan and breaking; or the syringe may be placed in a strainer which has been set in water for this purpose. In certain parts of the country the syringe may become coated from boiling in the hard water. These deposits can be prevented by wrapping the syringe and the needle in cloth or gauze before boiling.

Fig. 50. *Insulin should not be subjected to extremes of temperature, and insulin bottles not in use should be stored in the refrigerator, but freezing should be avoided.* The bottle of insulin that is being used can be kept at ordinary room temperature.

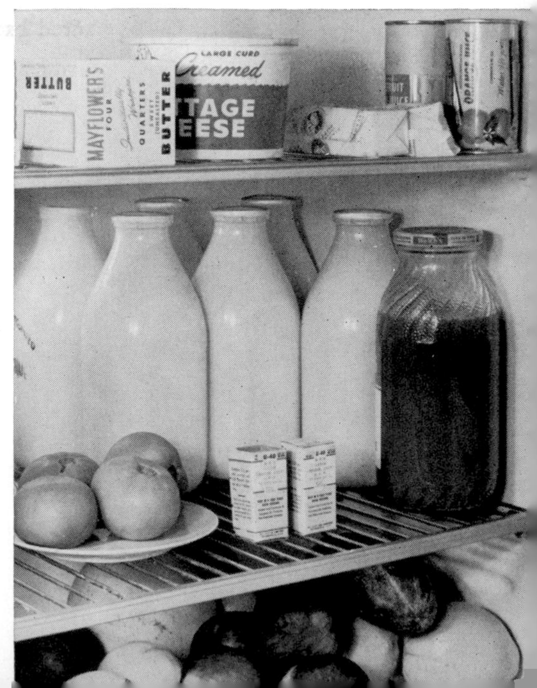

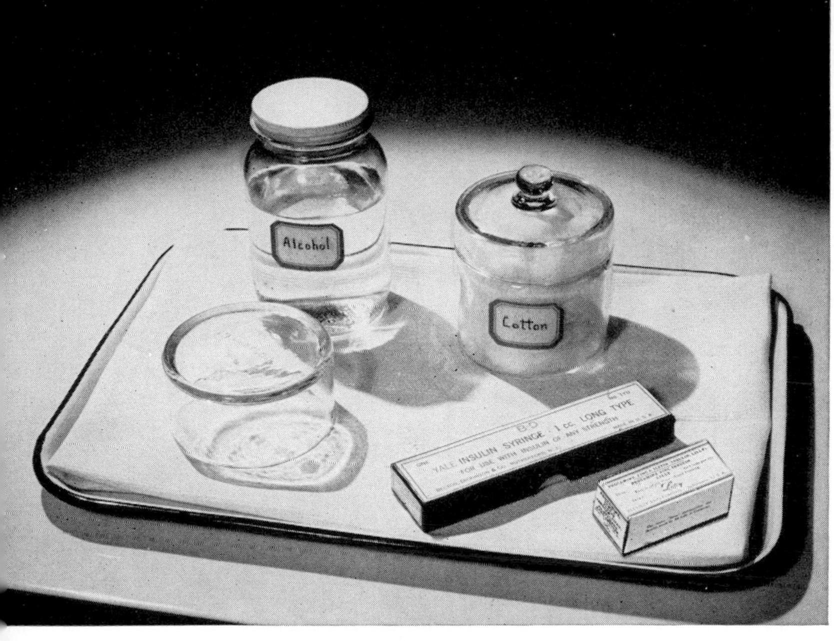

FIG 51. *The tray is left ready for the next injection.* The dish of cotton is covered, the bottle of alcohol closed, the dish for the alcohol turned upside down on the tray, the insulin bottle placed in the box, and the container for the syringe and the needle covered.

INJECTION OF INSULIN MIXTURES

Insulin mixtures are recommended in certain instances to meet individual needs more precisely. These mixtures are always determined and prescribed by the physician.

There are a few rules which apply in general to the use of insulin mixtures. The strengths of the two insulin preparations should be the same, both either U-40 or U-80 insulin. When larger doses are required, the total volume should be reduced whenever possible by using U-80 strength. (See Measurement and Strengths of Insulin Preparations, p. 100.)

Various combinations of insulins may be recommended. Unmodified insulin may be mixed with one of the following preparations of modified insulin: protamine zinc insulin, NPH insulin or lente insulin. When any of these mixtures is used it is essential that *unmodified insulin be drawn into the syringe first,* since the contents of the bottle of unmodified insulin should not be contaminated. This could easily change the action of this insulin preparation.

When lente insulin is used in a mixture with either semilente or ultralente insulin, there is no need for a special sequence in the preparation of the mixture, since these materials are all identical chemically.

PROCEDURE FOR THE INJECTION OF INSULIN MIXTURES

The following procedure is employed for the injection of insulin mixtures. The syringe, the needle and the two bottles of insulin are sterilized and prepared as described in Injection of Insulin (Figs. 15-26).

1. *The amount of air equal to the prescribed amount of modified insulin is drawn into the syringe* (Fig. 52).

2. *The air in the syringe is forced into the bottle of modified insulin* (Fig. 53).

3. *The needle is withdrawn* (Fig. 54).

4. *Then, as described in Figures 27-31, the prescribed amount of unmodified insulin is drawn into the syringe, and the needle is withdrawn from the bottle* (Fig. 55).

5. *The bottle of modified insulin is tipped upside down* so that the insulin is next to the stopper, and the needle of the syringe, which already contains the unmodified insulin, is inserted in the bottle of modified insulin. The plunger is allowed to rest against the hand so that it does not slip (Fig. 56).

6. *The prescribed amount of modified insulin is drawn into the syringe* in addition to the unmodified insulin already in the syringe (Fig. 57).

7. *The needle is withdrawn from the bottle of modified insulin* (Fig. 58).

8. *The syringe, containing the two insulins, is held upright,* the needle at the top, and the plunger is pulled down slightly until a small air bubble can be seen (Fig. 59).

9A, 9B. *The syringe is held level and tilted slowly* from one end to the other. In this way the air bubble rolls through the insulins and so they become mixed. This is done until the insulins are well mixed (Fig. 60).

10. *The air bubble is removed* from the syringe by again holding the syringe upright and pushing the plunger gently so that only the air bubble, but no insulin, is forced out (Fig. 61).

11. *The syringe, filled with the mixture of insulins, is ready for injection.* The method of injection is the same as that described in Injection of Insulin, Figures 32-42 (Fig. 62).

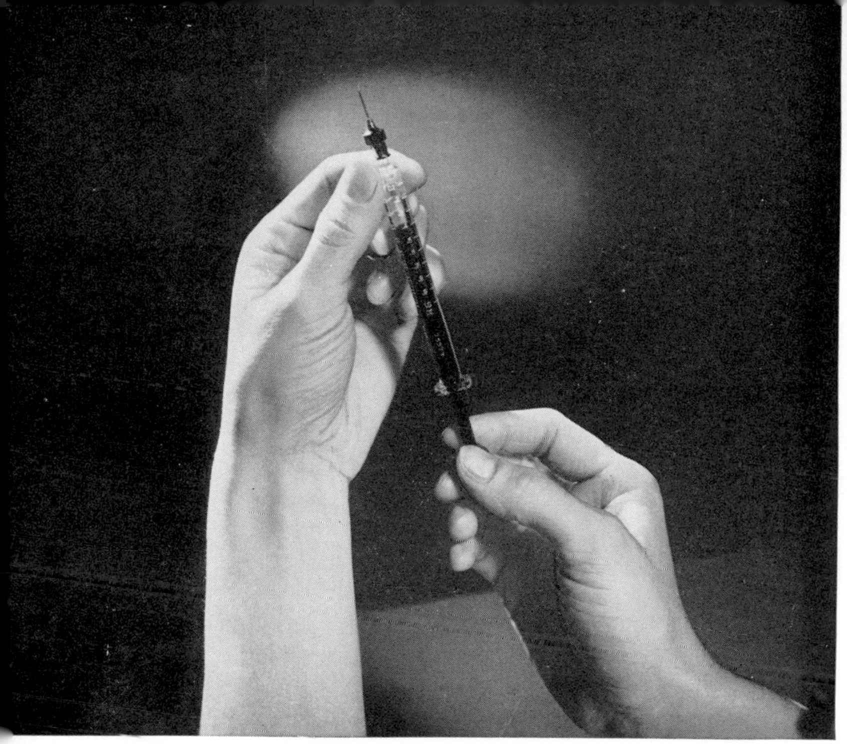

FIG. 52. *The amount of air equal to the prescribed amount of modified insulin is drawn into the syringe.*

FIG. 53. *The air in the syringe is forced into the bottle of modified insulin.*

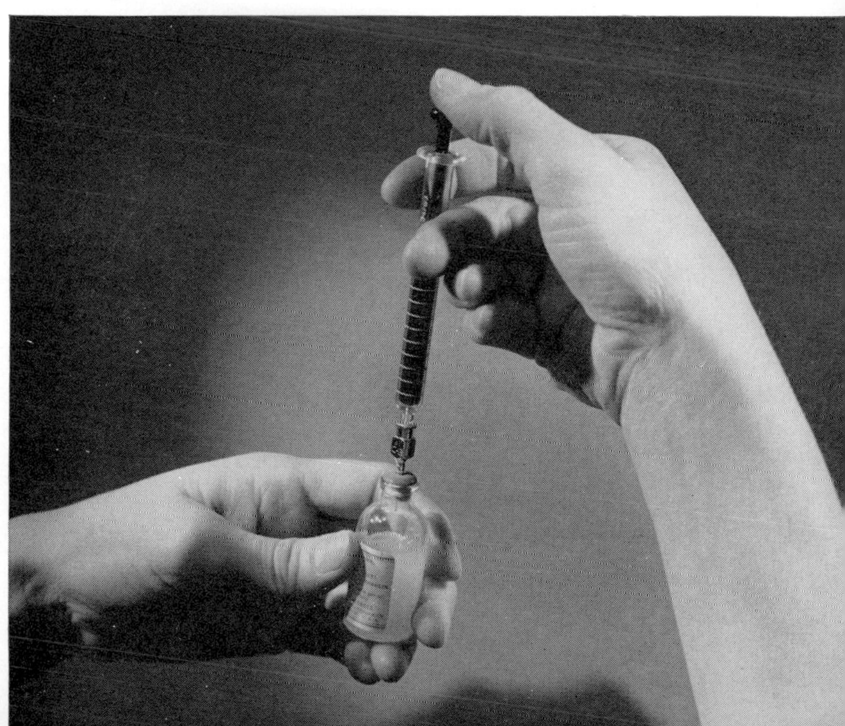

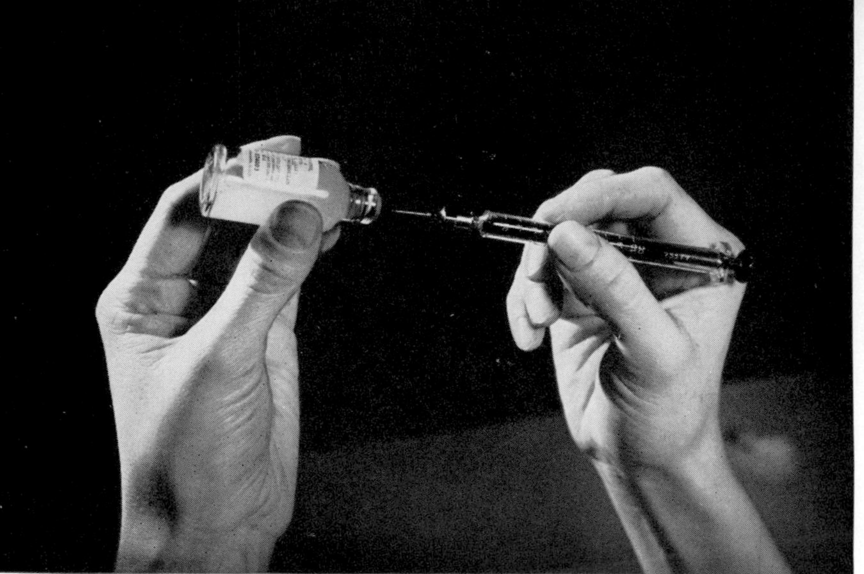

FIG. 54. *The needle is withdrawn.*

FIG. 55. *Then* (as described in Figs. 27 to 31) *the prescribed amount of unmodified insulin is drawn into the syringe, and the needle is withdrawn from the bottle.*

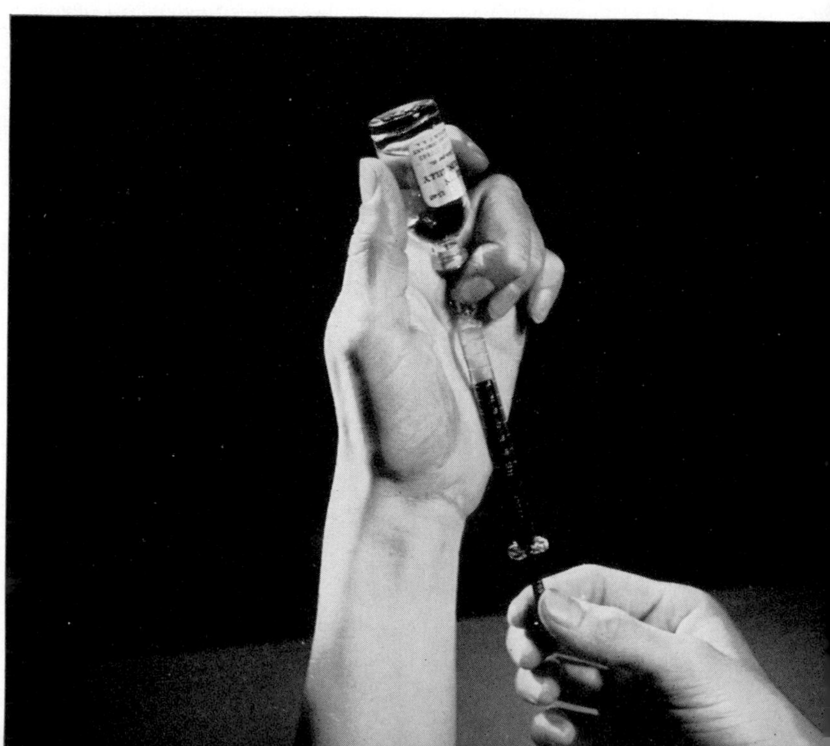

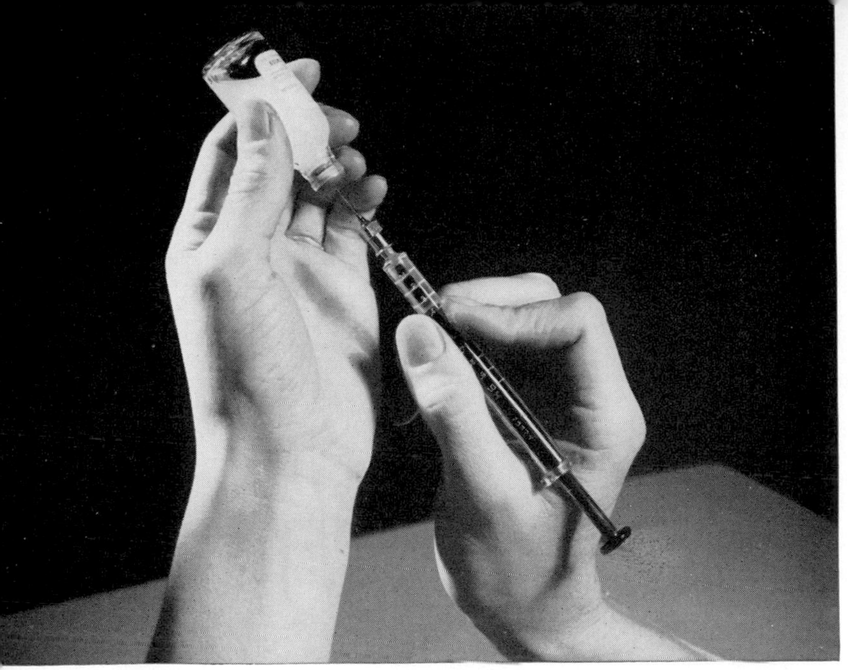

Fig. 56. *The bottle of modified insulin is tipped upside down* so that the insulin is next to the stopper, and the needle of the syringe which already contains the unmodified insulin is inserted in the bottle of modified insulin. The plunger is allowed to rest against the hand so that it does not slip.

Fig. 57. *The prescribed amount of modified insulin is drawn into the syringe* in addition to the unmodified insulin already in the syringe.

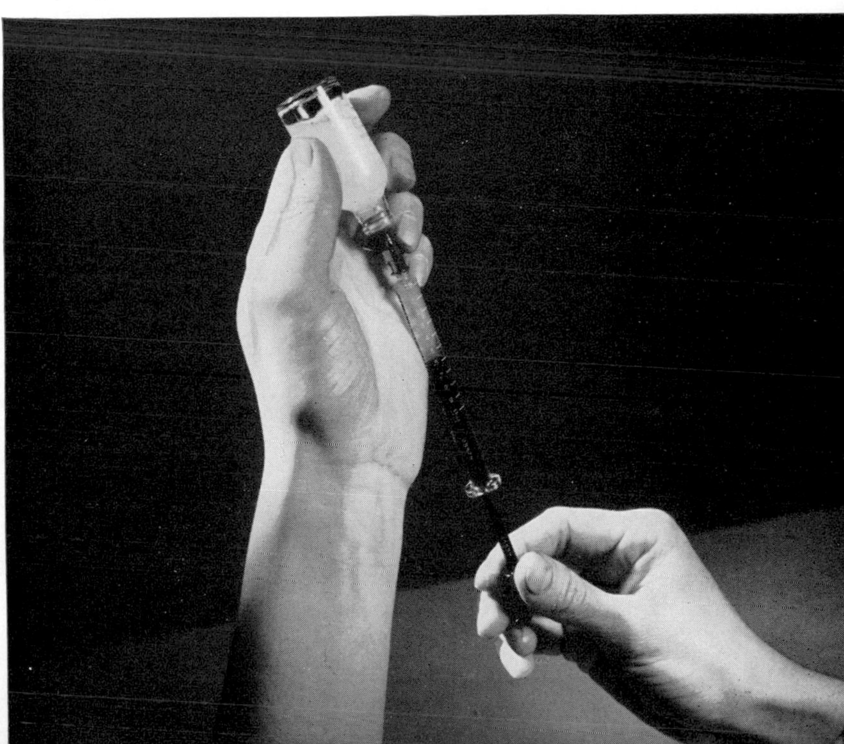

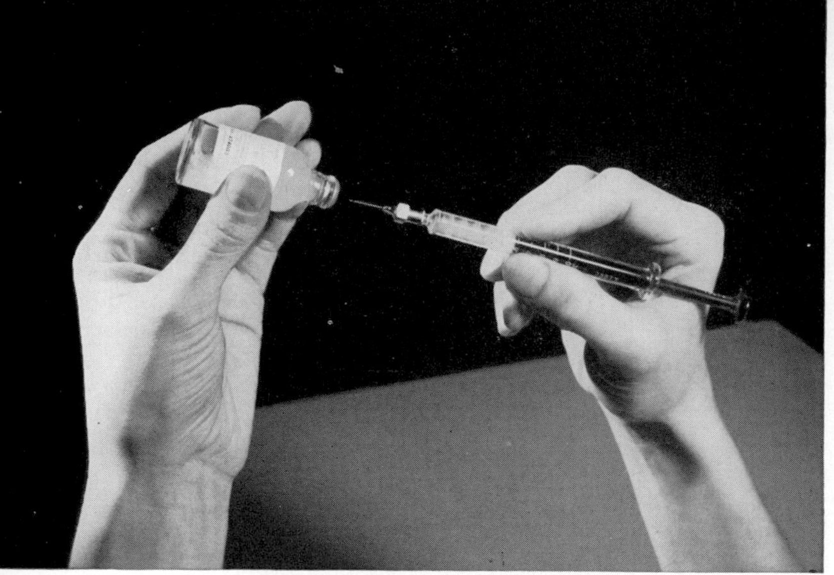

FIG. 58. *The needle is withdrawn from the bottle of modified insulin.*

FIG. 59. *The syringe, containing the two insulins, is held upright,* the needle at the top, and the plunger is pulled down slightly until a small air bubble can be seen.

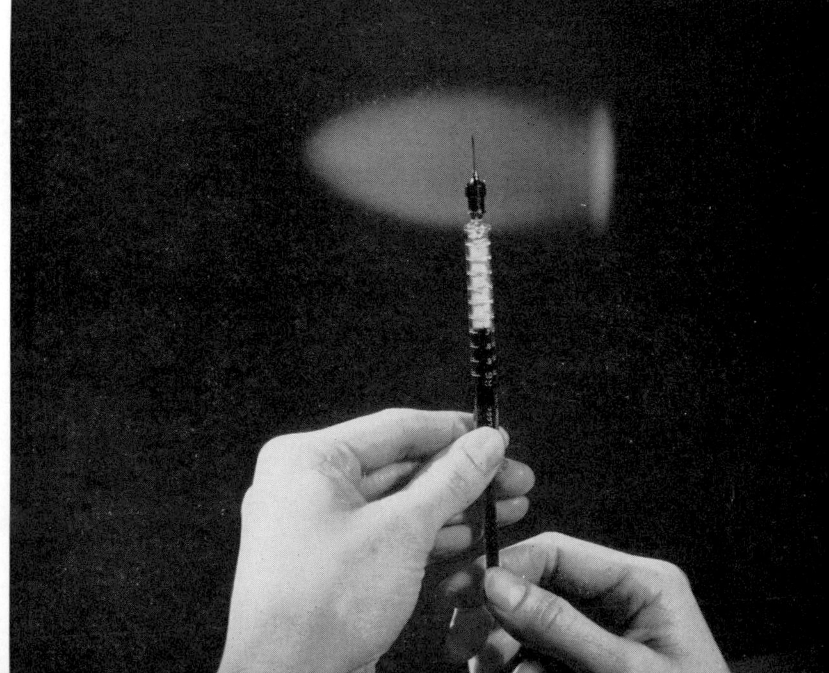

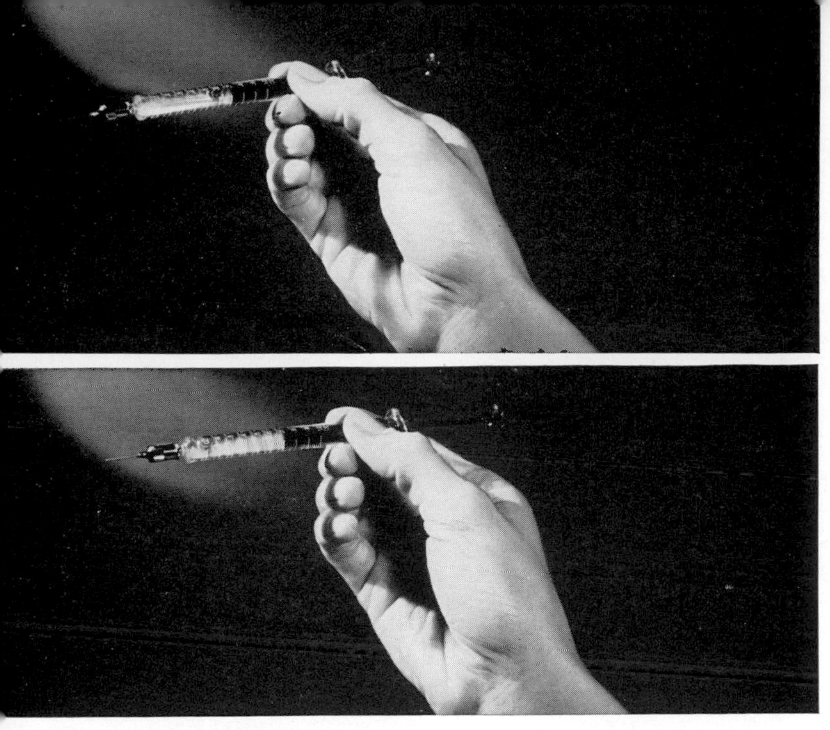

Fig. 60. *The syringe is held level and tilted slowly* from one end to the other. In this way the air bubble rolls through the insulins, and so they become mixed. This is done until the insulins are well mixed.

Fig. 61. *The air bubble is removed* from the syringe by again holding the syringe upright and pushing the plunger gently so that only the air bubble, but no insulin, is forced out.

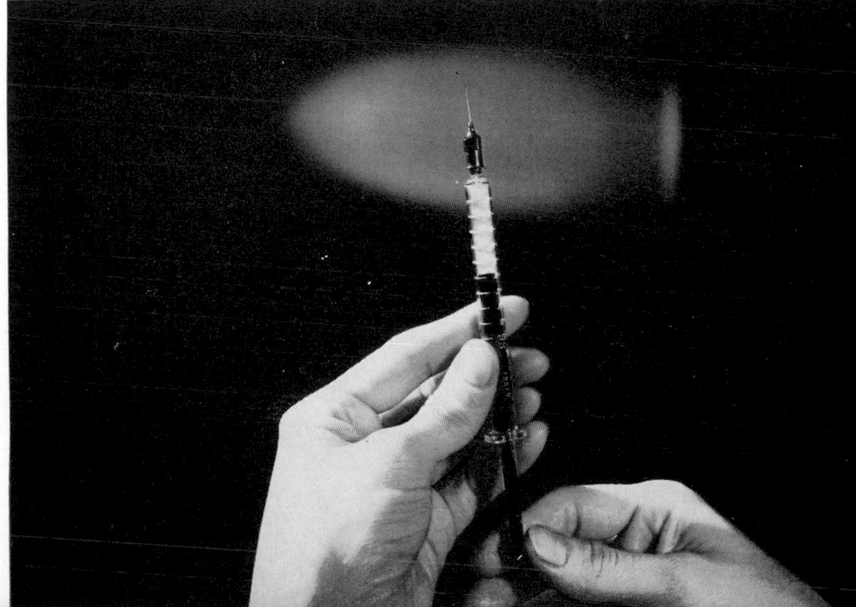

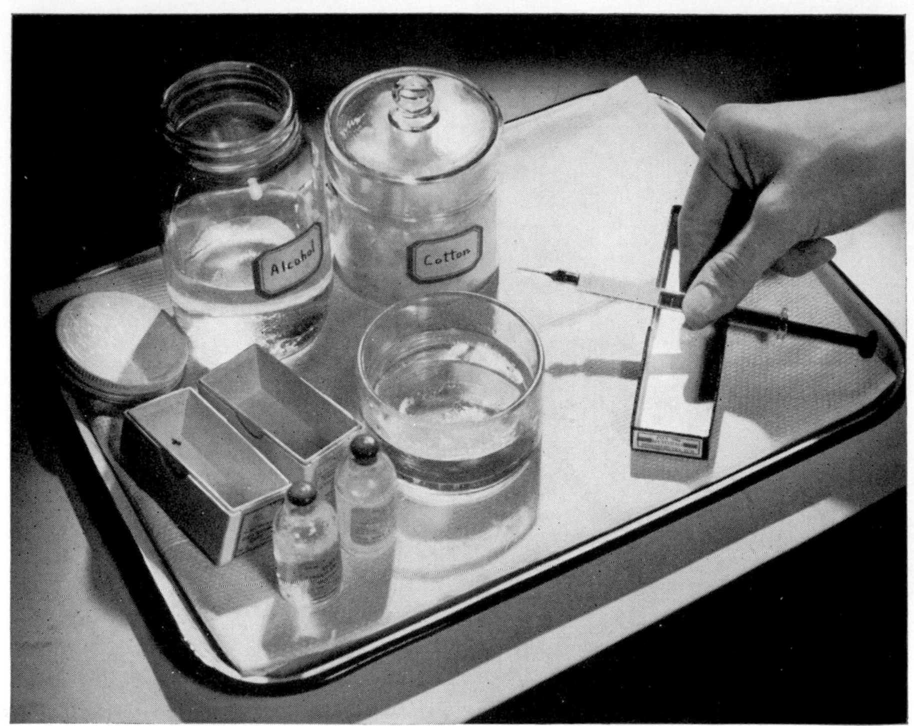

FIG. 62. *The syringe, filled with the mixture of insulin, is ready for injection.* The method of injection is the same as that described in Injection of Insulin (Figures 32 to 42).

INSULIN ALLERGY

Local reactions due to insulin allergy are encountered more often when treatment is first begun. Usually, they are manifested by small to large red areas at the site of injection and may be associated with itching and pain. These local reactions may appear soon after the insulin is injected or within a day or two, and they may persist for several days. In unusual instances there may be local or generalized hives (urticaria).

Insulin allergy usually results from a sensitivity to the protein substances contained in the insulin. When local reactions are mild, they frequently can be eliminated by one of several procedures. Daily injections may be continued, using smaller amounts of insulin until the reactions diminish and disappear. Some local reactions are due to superficial (intradermal) injections and may be eliminated by injecting the insulin deeper into the subcutaneous tissue. Often, the use of another type or brand of insulin, or of "special insulin" obtained from either beef or pork pancreas, will be helpful. In the event that these procedures are not effective, it may be necessary to employ a desensitization method whereby frequent injections of dilute solutions are given, gradually increasing the amount of insulin until the prescribed dosage can be tolerated. This should always be done under the supervision of the physician.

There have been instances where the alcohol used for purposes of sterilization has been responsible for the inflammation at the site of the injection. Under such circumstances some other means of sterilization should be employed.

At times there may be a gradual disappearance of fatty tissue under the skin at the site of injection, causing a depression or "dimpling." The exact cause of this is not known. Except for cosmetic reasons, there is no need for concern, but in such an event frequent injections in the same area should be avoided.

4. COMPLICATIONS OF DIABETES
INSULIN REACTIONS—HYPOGLYCEMIA
DIABETIC ACIDOSIS AND COMA

INSULIN REACTIONS
(Hypoglycemia)

When there is a correct balance between food and insulin, whether it is body insulin or body-and-bottle insulin, blood-sugar levels are kept within limits of safety and comfort, and the urine usually contains little or no sugar (Fig. 2). However, when insulin is present in excess, the balance between food and insulin becomes upset, and the blood sugar falls below the normal level (*hypo*—less than normal, *glycemia*—sugar in the blood). When this occurs, the terms "insulin reaction" or "insulin shock" are used to describe the series of events that may ensue. Insulin reactions may occur shortly after the injection of insulin, or many hours later, depending upon the type of insulin used (p. 90).

Hypoglycemia may occur occasionally with oral drug therapy (p. 141).

Signs and Symptoms of Insulin Reactions

An insulin reaction may affect the patient in any of the following ways: The feeling of sudden hunger or weakness, nervousness, usually with perspiration and often with trembling. Persistent headaches before meals, a feeling of drowsiness or nausea, or a sensation of numbness or tingling around the mouth or in the fingers. The patient may laugh or cry, become anxious and confused, or become dizzy with blurred or double vision. In some instances, patients have been known to become disoriented, lose the power of speech, get excited and to develop a staggering gait. Unconsciousness may result if an insulin reaction continues untreated (Table 14).

Causes of Insulin Reactions

As already explained, insulin reactions occur when, as a result of too much insulin for the amount of sugar in the body, the blood sugar falls below normal levels (Fig. 2). An excessive amount of insulin may be taken as a result of incorrect measurement. Often, reactions may occur during the early period of treatment when less insulin is required as the patient's carbohydrate tolerance improves. The patient may have an insulin reaction when he is unable to, or does not, take his prescribed diet (meals and intermediate feedings), or when there is a loss of food due to vomiting or diarrhea. Often, the blood sugar will fall to low levels when the intervals between meals are prolonged or when a meal or an intermediate feeding is omitted.

Another consideration is the amount of exercise taken. A moderate amount of exercise is desirable, since it helps to burn sugar in the body; but when more exercise than planned for is taken, the blood sugar may fall to low levels. Additional carbohydrate should be taken before an unusual amount of exercise, such as bowling, tennis, walking or dancing, to help prevent the possibility of an insulin reaction. (See Exercise, p. 167.)

Caution should be taken to avoid an insulin reaction when driving a motor vehicle or when engaged in a hazardous occupation, particularly one that requires working with machinery or at a high elevation. It may be well to have the diabetes so regulated that small amounts of sugar will be present in the urine at times to ensure against the occurrence of an insulin reaction.

Treatment for an Insulin Reaction

Treatment for an insulin reaction consists in supplying the body with carbohydrate to counterbalance the fall in blood sugar. A concentrated form of sugar is given. This may be granulated or lump sugar, candy, jam or jelly, which will be absorbed rapidly by the body, thus raising the level of the blood sugar. Fruit juices may also be used for this purpose. Usually from 20 to 25 grams of carbohydrate are required to overcome an insulin reaction, or the amount contained in 4 teaspoonfuls of granulated sugar, or 4 lumps of sugar, or in the juice of 2 oranges. If the reaction continues, the same amount of carbohydrate should be repeated at intervals of 10 to 15 minutes.

When unmodified insulin is used the reaction develops rapidly and usually can be overcome in a short period of time. With the use of the slow- and intermediate-acting insulins a reaction develops more slowly, as a rule, and takes longer to overcome. Therefore, treatment for this type of reaction requires, in addition to concentrated carbohydrate, other foods that are absorbed more slowly, such as a glass of milk with a slice of bread, or crackers or cereal instead of the slice of bread.

It is advisable to remain quiet until an insulin reaction is over, so that the sugar that has been taken will be used, not for body activity but for raising the level of the blood sugar.

Responsible members of the family should know how to treat an insulin reaction, for at times the patient may suffer confusion or unconsciousness. When unconsciousness exists it is wise to call a physician at once so that he may inject sugar in the form of glucose into the vein. Sugar should not be given in liquid form when the patient is unconscious, as it may cause choking. Instead, until the physician arrives, sugar in dry form, such as granulated sugar, may be placed under the tongue or inside the cheek, where it will be absorbed.

Identification Card

An insulin reaction or acidosis (see following paragraph for acidosis) may result in mental confusion or, in extreme cases, unconsciousness or coma.

The patient then would be unable to care for himself and would depend upon those near him for help. Therefore, to ensure proper care at all times, an identification card or tag* should be carried which contains the following information:

Statement of Disease—Diabetes

Patient's name, address and telephone number

Name, address and telephone number of physician or institution treating patient

Food prescription—carbohydrate, protein and fat

Insulin prescription—number of units and kind of insulin

or

Oral drug—kind and amount

Request that sugar or candy be given immediately, and that a physician be called if there is no improvement within 15 minutes.

DIABETIC ACIDOSIS AND COMA

Diabetic acidosis and coma are the most important of the acute complications of diabetes.

Acidosis, a serious consequence of uncontrolled diabetes, results when sugar cannot be utilized and fat is called upon to supply the body's need for energy. Under these conditions there is a limit to the amount of fat the body can burn completely. When this limit is reached certain substances, diacetic acid and acetone (ketone bodies), which are formed in the process of the burning of fat, accumulate in the body more quickly than the body can rid itself of them. This accumulation of diacetic acid and acetone in the body is called acidosis or ketosis. There are several conditions that can cause the development of diabetic acidosis.

Causes of Acidosis

The most common causes of diabetic acidosis and coma are acute infections such as pneumonia, carbuncles, severe infections of the extremities and intestinal disorders. Acidosis also may develop when, in certain instances, insulin is omitted or when the prescribed treatment is ignored or abandoned. When immediate intensive treatment is not given, acidosis can become more severe and progress to diabetic coma. Neglect of immediate treatment for diabetic coma can result in death (Table 14).

Signs and Symptoms of Acidosis

Members of the family, as well as the patient, should be able to recognize *the signs and symptoms of acidosis* so that a physician may be summoned as soon as this condition is suspected. When acidosis is present the patient appears to be ill and may become drowsy or very irritable. One is thirsty, as a rule, with no appetite. Vomiting may occur, and cramps or pains in the abdomen, the arms or the legs. The skin is dry and cold to the touch, and the face is flushed. Vision is often

* **Note:** Information concerning identification cards or tags can be obtained from the American Diabetes Association, Inc., the physician or the institution treating the patient.

dimmed or blurred, and the eyeballs are soft. There may be a sweet, "fruity" odor from the breath. The patient often complains of not having enough air ("air hunger") and breathes deeply. Urine tests show the presence of diacetic acid and acetone in addition to large amounts of sugar. (For directions for these tests, see Chap. 6.) When acidosis is mild the patient is awake but may feel drowsy. As the condition becomes more severe, and coma is approaching, the patient becomes more drowsy, and eventually unconscious (Table 14).

Care of the Patient with Acidosis

Acidosis, a forerunner of diabetic coma, should be treated early and vigorously. The services of a physician should be obtained as soon as possible. Insulin is of prime importance in the treatment of acidosis and is always required for this condition.

Constant attention should be given to the patient with acidosis until he is under the care of a physician. Until medical care is obtained the following directions should be carried out:

Fluid in the form of clear broth, tea or coffee should be taken frequently unless the patient is vomiting. A specimen of urine should be obtained, if possible, so that it may be tested for sugar and acetone (Chap. 6). When there is fever, the patient should stay in bed and keep warm until the physician arrives. It may be necessary to wrap him in blankets or to use heating pads or hot-water bottles that have been covered to avoid body burns.

Severe acidosis or diabetic coma makes hospitalization mandatory.

Table 14. Comparison of Clinical Features of Insulin Reactions and Diabetic Coma*

Clinical Feature	Insulin Reaction	Diabetic Coma
Onset	Sudden or gradual (minutes to hours)	Slow (days)
Causes	Delayed mealtime Omission of meal Excessive exercise Insulin overdosage	Neglect of treatment Intercurrent disease Acute infections
Symptoms	Nervousness Weakness Sweating Hunger Blurred or double vision Abnormal behavior	Thirst Headache Irritability Nausea Vomiting Abdominal pain Dim vision Constipation Shortness of breath
Signs	Pallor Shallow respiration Sweating Pulse normal Eyeballs normal Unconsciousness Convulsions	Florid face Air hunger Loud, labored breathing Dry skin Rapid pulse Soft eyeballs Acetone breath Drowsiness Loss of consciousness
Urinalysis:		
Sugar	Usually absent, especially in second voided specimen	Positive
Acetone	Negative	Positive
Response to Treatment	Rapid; occasionally delayed	Slow

* Adapted from Diabetes Mellitus, Eli Lilly and Company.

5. ORAL HYPOGLYCEMIC AGENTS

EVER since insulin was discovered there has been a constant hope that an oral preparation for the treatment of diabetes might be found, thereby eliminating the necessity for hypodermic injections. Now, for some, this hope has been realized.

The story of oral drugs portrays another exciting series of events in the history of diabetes and its treatment. Early in 1942 the therapeutic effects of derivatives of sulfanilamide were being investigated in France by M. Janbon and his associates at the Medical School of Montpellier. It was found that this drug produced, in certain patients, symptoms and signs resembling hypoglycemia (low blood-sugar).

Later, that same year, this information was presented to the French physiologist Auguste Loubatière, also in Montpellier, at the Institute of Biology. He not only confirmed that hypoglycemic effects were produced by this "sulfa" drug, but also noted that when the pancreata of the animals being studied were removed, this drug no longer produced a lowering of sugar levels in the blood. As a result of further investigation it was concluded that the presence of some insulin-secreting cells in the pancreas (beta cells in the islands of Langerhans) was essential for the successful action of this drug with regard to the lowering of the blood sugar.

Meanwhile, other investigators became interested in the "sulfa" drugs, and, from the year 1947 to 1955, studies were carried on in many countries. In 1955 intensive clinical trials were begun on humans, not only in France, Germany, Denmark and Argentina but in the United States and Canada as well. The two "sulfa" drugs used in these clinical trials were carbutamide (BZ55) and tolbutamide (Orinase). Carbutamide was withdrawn because of untoward effects in a small number of patients. Tolbutamide, on the other hand, became widely accepted for the treatment of the patient with stable, adult-type diabetes in the middle or older age group.

The oral hypoglycemic agents come from the same chemical family—the sulfonylurea compounds—as do the famous "sulfa" drugs. Although chemically related to the sulfa drugs used in the treatment of certain infections, these hypoglycemic agents have no such antibacterial properties. The exact mechanism of the action is not fully understood, but it is believed that they stimulate the secretion of insulin by the beta cells in the pancreas.

Currently, in addition to tolbutamide (Orinase*), there are three other sulfonylurea compounds available for the treatment of diabetes, namely chlorpropamide (Diabinese†), acetohexa-

* Trademark of The Upjohn Company.

† Trademark of Pfizer Laboratories.

mide (Dymelor*) and tolazamide (Tolinase†).

In the interim, another oral hypoglycemic agent, phenformin (DBI‡), became available. Phenformin is not a sulfonylurea, but belongs to the chemical group called biguanides. It is completely unrelated chemically to the sulfonylurea compounds and its blood-sugar-lowering action is entirely different.

The two groups of oral hypoglycemic agents, the sulfonylureas and the biguanides, are discussed further in this chapter.

The advisability of using oral agents, the selection of a particular drug, and the amount to be taken should always be determined by the physician. In any event, the patient must realize that every rule involved in the total treatment needs to be followed with meticulous care, just as with insulin therapy.

Although the success of therapy with oral agents usually may be anticipated by the physician, there are instances when they are not effective from the start. This is referred to as "primary failure." There are other times when, after weeks, months or even years, there is unfavorable response to the oral compounds. This unfavorable response is referred to as "secondary failure." In such cases insulin therapy becomes necessary.

As a rule, the oral hypoglycemic agents are especially successful in patients with mild, maturity-onset diabetes—acquired when the patient was over forty years old. Persons are considered responsive to oral therapy when they are symptom-free, with little or no sugar in the urine and when blood-sugar levels are within reasonably normal limits.

The oral hypoglycemic agents are not indicated for the treatment of children and most young adults; for the treatment of severe diabetes when large amounts of insulin are required for control; or for "unstable" or so-called brittle diabetes except under special circumstances.

There is general agreement that oral hypoglycemic agents should not be used when the diabetes can be controlled with the use of diet alone. The importance of adherence to the prescribed diet cannot be overemphasized.

The action of oral hypoglycemic agents is entirely different from that of insulin and, therefore, they are never to be regarded as a substitute for insulin whenever it is required.

THE SULFONYLUREA COMPOUNDS

There are presently available four sulfonylurea compounds, namely, Orinase (tolbutamide), Diabinese (chlorpropamide), Dymelor (acetohexamide) and Tolinase (tolazamide). Following are descriptions of each of these, including shape, color, size and duration

* Trademark of Eli Lilly Company.
† Trademark of The Upjohn Company.
‡ Trademark of U. S. Vitamin & Pharmaceutical Corporation.

TABLE 15. ORAL HYPOGLYCEMIC AGENTS

AGENT (Drug)	DESCRIPTION			DURATION OF ACTION
	SHAPE	COLOR	SIZE (Milligrams)	
Sulfonylureas				
Orinase (tolbutamide) (The Upjohn Company)	Round tablet	White	500	6 to 12 hours
Diabinese (chlorpropamide) (Pfizer Laboratories)	"D" shaped tablet	Blue Blue	250 100	up to 60 hours
Dymelor (acetohexamide) (Eli Lilly Company)	Capsule-shaped tablet	White Yellow	250 500	12 to 24 hours
Tolinase (tolazamide) (The Upjohn Company)	Round tablet	White White	100 250	12 to 24 hours
Biguanides				
DBI (phenformin) (U.S. Vitamin & Pharmaceutical Corporation)	Round tablet	White	25	4 to 6 hours
DBI-TD (phenformin–timed disintegration) (U.S. Vitamin & Pharmaceutical Corporation)	Capsule	Blue and white	50	8 to 12 hours

of action. This description is summarized in Table 15.

Orinase is prepared in a round, white tablet containing 500 milligrams. The duration of its action is about 6 to 12 hours. As a rule, this agent is most effective when taken twice daily, usually before the morning and evening meal (Table 15).

Diabinese is prepared in a "D"-shaped blue tablet. There are two sizes, 100 and 250 milligrams. Its action is more prolonged than that of the other sulfonylurea compounds, lasting up to about 60 hours. Usually, it is prescribed to be taken once a day (Table 15).

Dymelor is prepared in a capsule-shaped tablet, in two sizes and colors. The 250-milligram tablet is white, and the 500-milligram tablet is yellow. The duration of the action of Dymelor ranges from 12 to 24 hours. It may be prescribed to be taken once or twice a day (Table 15).

Tolinase is prepared in a round, white tablet. There are two sizes, 100 milligrams and 250 milligrams. The action of this preparation lasts about 12 to 24 hours and it is prescribed to be taken once or twice a day (Table 15).

THE BIGUANIDES (PHENFORMIN)

It was not until 1957 that the biguanides (phenformin) were used in the treatment of diabetes. This group of drugs is distinctly different from and unrelated in chemical structure to the sulfonylurea compounds. Phenformin, unlike the sulfonylurea group, has nothing to do with stimulating or increasing the amount of insulin supplied by the beta cells in the pancreas. Although the exact nature of its blood-sugar-lowering action is not clearly understood, phenformin seems to lower the blood sugar in the presence of insulin, either endogenous (body insulin) or exogenous (injected or "bottle" insulin).

In general, this agent has been used for certain patients with "adult-onset" or "maturity-onset" diabetes. At times it is used in conjunction with insulin or sulfonylurea compounds to achieve better diabetic control, especially with "unstable" or "brittle" diabetes.

The phenformin marketed in the United States is called DBI and is available in two forms: DBI is prepared in a round, white tablet containing 25 milligrams, the action of which lasts 4 to 6 hours (Table 15). DBI-TD (timed disintegration) is available in a blue and white capsule containing 50 milligrams. The action of DBI-TD lasts from about 8 to 12 hours (Table 15).

As with the other oral agents, success in treatment depends upon strict adherence to the diet. DBI should not be used without continuous medical supervision.

GENERAL CONSIDERATIONS

There are significant general considerations in regard to therapy with oral hypoglycemic agents that deserve emphasis.

Therapy is always determined by the physician and is based on the needs of the individual patient.

The use of oral compounds is not indicated when adequate control of the diabetes can be achieved with dietary management alone. This is particularly true in the case of those people in the older age groups who are overweight and have mild diabetes, and for whom weight reduction is essential.

Oral therapy does not lessen in any way the need for strict adherence to every measure concerned with total treatment—diet, body weight, exercise, personal hygiene and the avoidance of infection. In addition, urine tests for sugar (p. 146) need to be done regularly—and also, when indicated, the test for acetone (p. 163).

The division of the total food in the diet should be so arranged in meals as to provide an equal distribution of carbohydrate throughout the day. The number of intermediate feedings and the times when they are to be taken are an individual matter determined by the physician.

The patient should be familiar with the signs and symptoms of hypoglycemia even though this may seldom occur if at all. In the event of its occurrence, however, one needs to counteract it immediately, as with insulin therapy (p. 136).

Occasionally there may be so-called *side-effects* with the use of oral agents. Usually these are not of a serious nature and ordinarily can be overcome by adjustments in therapy. The side-effects may consist in gastro-intestinal disturbances, headache and/or allergic skin manifestations. The gastro-intestinal disturbances include conditions such as nausea, epigastric fullness and heartburn. Headache appears to be related to the size of the dose and frequently disappears when the dosage is reduced or adjusted. Allergic skin manifestations such as itching and urticaria (hives) usually are transient. In addition to the side-effects just described, the use of DBI (phenformin) may cause an unpleasant, metallic or bitter taste in the mouth, nausea or vomiting, loss of appetite, and, in some instances, diarrhea. Sometimes these can be overcome with adjustments in the dosage. In the event that side-effects persist with any of the oral drugs, total withdrawal may be necessary.

A peculiar reaction to alcohol may occur in a small percentage of persons taking sulfonylurea compounds, in which case the use of alcohol is not recommended. This reaction may occur within minutes after the ingestion of even a small amount of an alcoholic beverage and can last as long as an hour or more. The usual symptoms include a feeling of warmth, with "flushing" of the face, and/or a throbbing headache, nausea, giddiness, shortness of breath and fast heart beat. Photosensitivity reactions (sensitivity to light) may also occur.

The action of oral hypoglycemic agents is entirely different from that of insulin and, therefore, they are never to be regarded as a substitute for insulin whenever insulin is required. Although oral agents do not cure diabetes or replace insulin, they are of greatest value in the convenience they provide by freeing patients from the routine of daily insulin injections. Much has been learned about the oral agents in a relatively short period of time. Of no little importance is the stimulation of further research in the entire field of diabetes. Much can be anticipated as additional knowledge is acquired.

6. BLOOD AND URINE TESTS

THERE are certain blood and urine tests that determine the diagnosis of diabetes and guide the treatment. The presence of sugar in the urine, regardless of the amount, usually denotes diabetes. The diagnosis is confirmed when blood-sugar levels are found to be elevated (Fig. 2).

BLOOD TESTS

Often, a single blood-sugar determination will furnish sufficient information for making a definite diagnosis of diabetes. However, when a single blood test does not furnish necessary information, a further test—called a glucose-tolerance test—usually is carried out. The procedure for the glucose-tolerance test is as follows: The patient is given a specified amount of glucose (sugar), and then blood examinations are made at definite intervals over a period of 2 to 3 hours to determine blood-sugar levels. Urine tests are also taken at the same time. On occasion, other tests are necessary to make a definite diagnosis.

URINE TESTS

There are several tests for determining the presence of sugar in the urine. The procedures for these are easy, but it should be remembered that tests must be done correctly, for no test is reliable if performed improperly. Urine tests can and should be done by the patient according to the schedule set by the physician.

Among the more popular urine tests for sugar are Benedict's Test (p. 148), Clinitest (p. 155), Tes-Tape (p. 161), and Clinistix (p. 162). The directions for these tests are easily followed, and the equipment can be obtained readily. They will serve the patient in following his progress and also are a necessary guide in treatment. The results of the tests which are reported to the physician will indicate the need for redistribution of food in the diet or for readjustment of the dosage of insulin or oral drug. Often, when insulin therapy is used in treatment, the physician will prefer that there be small amounts of sugar in the urine, at times, to ensure against the occurrence of insulin reactions.

The control of the diabetes often is disrupted during the course of certain complications, especially acute infections and gastro-intestinal upsets (vomiting and diarrhea). Therefore, when any of these conditions are present it is necessary to test the urine more frequently and report to the physician should the diabetes become uncontrolled.

When diabetes continues to remain uncontrolled, as evidenced by the presence of large amounts of sugar in the urine, the test for acetone should be done (pp. 163 and 164). When the test results show that acetone is present in the urine, the patient should notify the physician (Chap. 4).

There are times when the physician wishes to calculate the total amount of sugar spilled in the urine over a period of 24 hours. The directions for collecting a 24-hour specimen of urine are given below.

DIRECTIONS FOR COLLECTING A 24-HOUR SPECIMEN OF URINE

Equipment Needed. Clean, tightly covered container sufficiently large to hold entire collection of urine. Utensil for measuring the amount of urine collected. Clean bottle, which contains 3 to 4 ounces, to be used for the sample of the 24-hour specimen of urine.

Collecting the Specimen. The collection of urine is started the day before the visit to the physician to allow 24 hours for the collection. On that day the first specimen is not saved, as the collection of urine starts with the second passing of urine. All urine passed during that day and night, and including the first specimen passed next morning, comprises the 24-hour collection required. After the total amount of urine has been measured (pints or quarts), a bottled 3- to 4-ounce sample of this collection of urine is taken to the physician for analysis. The sample specimen should be labeled to indicate the patient's name and the total amount of the urine collected.

BENEDICT'S TEST FOR SUGAR IN THE URINE

PREPARATION

1.* *A tray set up with the necessary equipment is a convenience to the patient* The articles necessary for the test for sugar in the urine are: a metal or enamel household measuring cup, a container for collecting the specimen of urine, Benedict's solution,† a test tube, a medicine dropper, a teaspoon, a small glass or cup to serve as a stand for the test tube, a test-tube holder, or a paper napkin or paper towel folded for this purpose, and a clock (Fig. 63).

PROCEDURE

2. *Measure 5 cubic centimeters of Benedict's solution.* A teaspoonful measures this amount (Fig. 64).

3. *Pour the contents of the teaspoon into the test tube,* holding the tip of the teaspoon against the inside of the test tube (Fig. 65).

4. *Fill the medicine dropper with urine* (Fig. 66).

5. *Add 8 drops of the urine from the medicine dropper to the Benedict's solution in the test tube* (Fig. 67).

6. *Mix the urine and the Benedict's solution by tipping the test tube 3 or 4 times.* A finger is placed over the opening of the test tube so that the contents are not spilled (Fig. 68).

7. *Place the test tube with its contents in a cup of bubbling, boiling water.* Look at the time on the clock (Fig 69).

8. *Remove the test tube from the boiling water after 5 minutes.* A holder should be used to remove the hot test tube from the cup to protect the fingers, and the test tube should be placed in the small glass (Fig. 70).

9. *The color of the solution in the test tube shows the amount of sugar in the urine* (Plate 6).

10. *Notice the color of the solution in the test tube.* The color may be recorded with crayons on a special chart (Fig. 71).

11. Wash the articles on the tray after completing the test so that they may be ready for the next test. The stopper is placed back on the bottle of Benedict's solution. The cup, the container for urine and the small glass to hold the test tube are turned upside down on the tray (Fig. 72).

---

* The numbers refer to the pictures that follow.

† Benedict's qualitative solution can be obtained at a drugstore. It contains the following ingredients:

Copper sulfate (pure crystallized)	17.3 Gr.
Sodium or potassium citrate	173.0 Gr.
Sodium carbonate, crystallized	200.0 Gr.
Distilled water, to make	1000.0 cc.

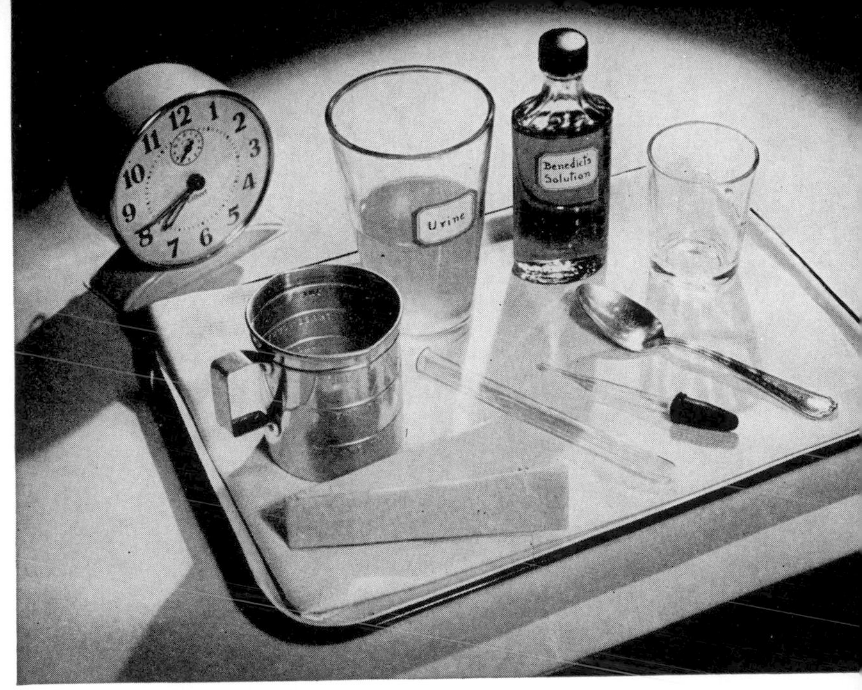

Fig. 63. *A tray set up with the necessary equipment is a convenience to the patient.* The articles necessary for the test for sugar in the urine are: a metal or enamel household measuring cup, a container for collecting the specimen of urine, Benedict's solution, a test tube, a medicine dropper, a teaspoon, a small glass or cup to serve as a stand for the test tube, a test-tube holder or a paper napkin or paper towel folded for this purpose, and a clock.

Fig. 64. *Measure 5 cubic centimeters of Benedict's solution.* A teaspoonful measures this amount.

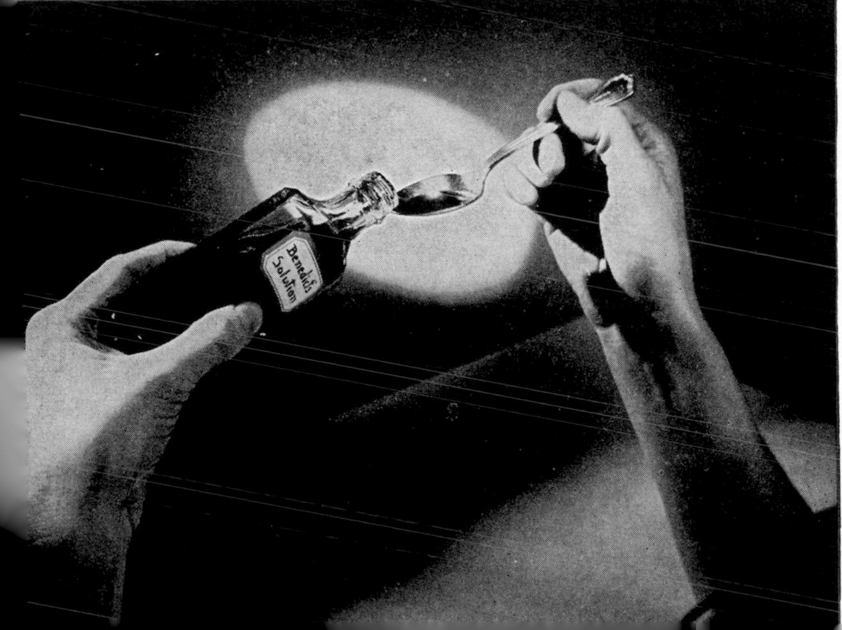

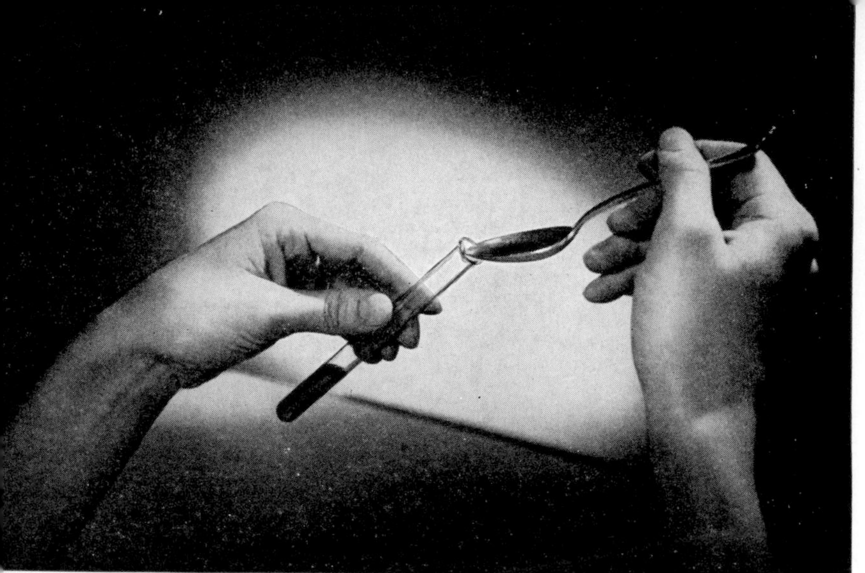

Fig. 65. *Pour the contents of the teaspoon into the test tube,* holding the tip of the teaspoon against the inside of the test tube.

Fig. 66. *Fill the medicine dropper with urine.*

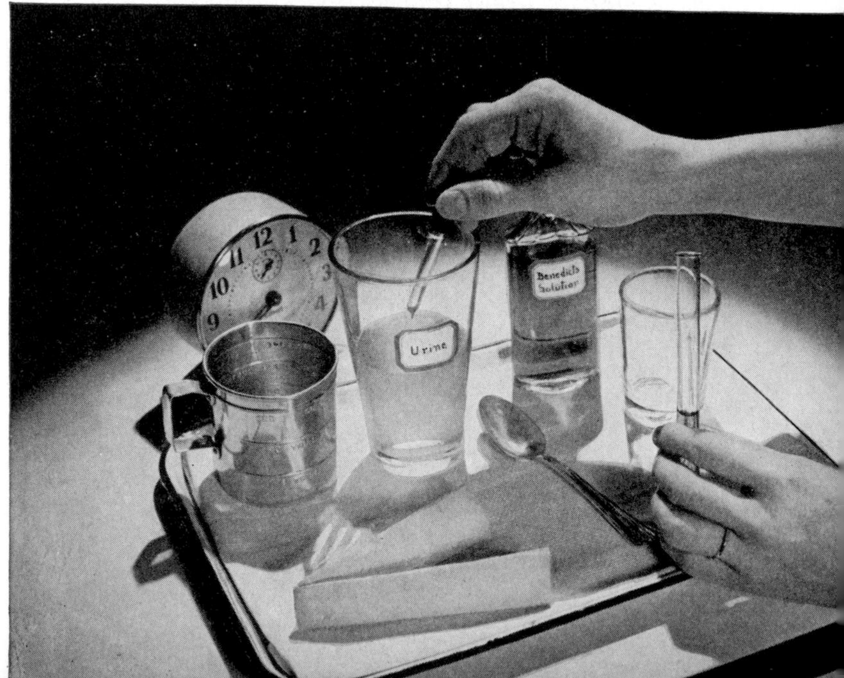

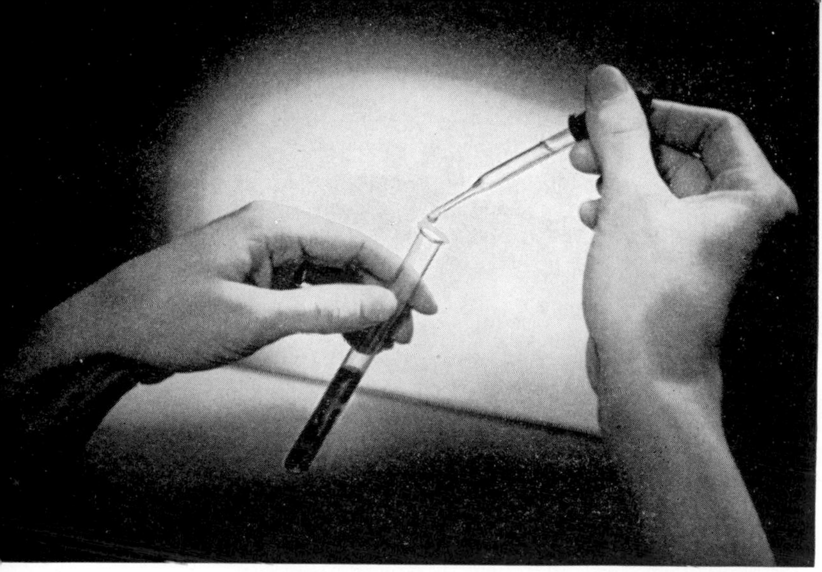

FIG. 67. *Add 8 drops of the urine from the medicine dropper to the Benedict's solution in the test tube.*

FIG. 68. *Mix the urine and the Benedict's solution* by tipping the test tube 3 or 4 times. A finger is placed over the opening of the test tube so that the contents are not spilled.

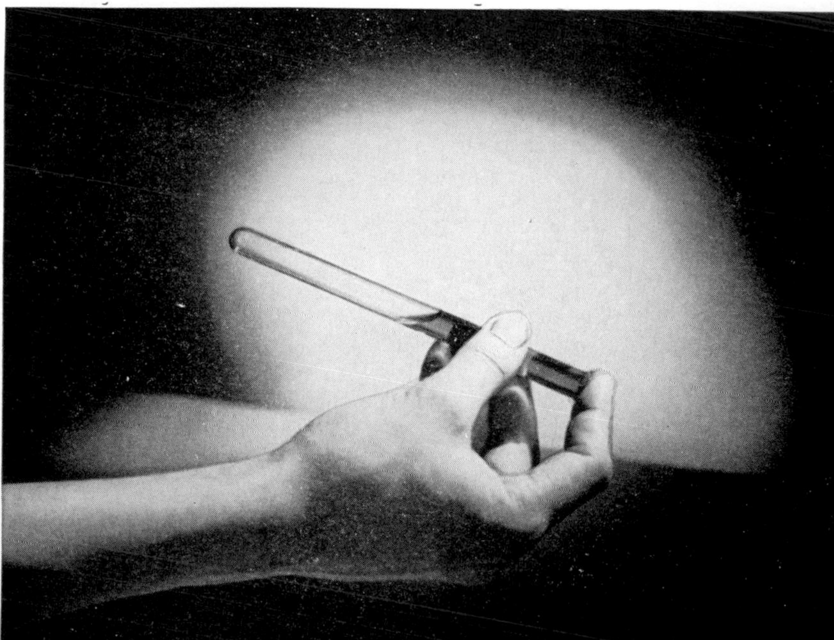

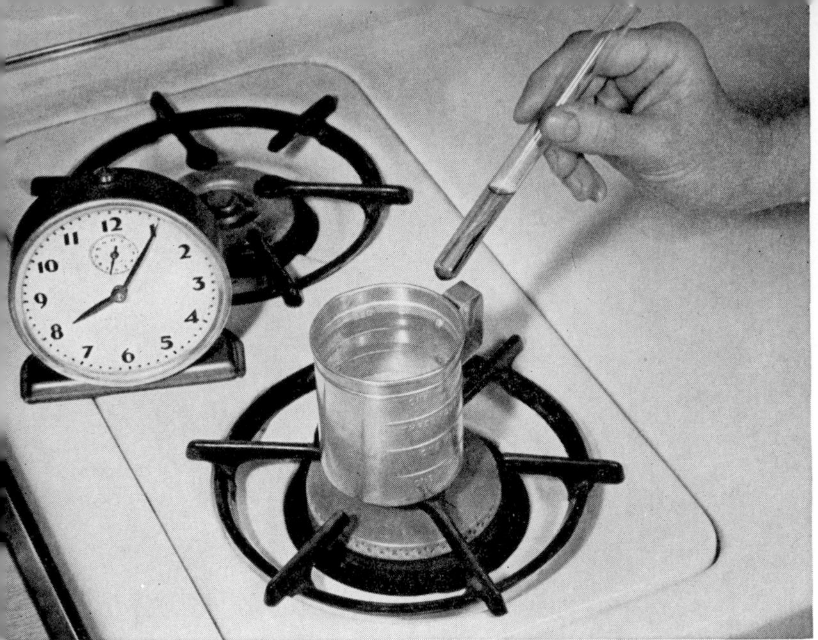

Fig. 69. *Place the test tube with its contents in a cup of bubbling, boiling water.* Look at the time on the clock.

Fig. 70. *Remove the test tube from the boiling water after 5 minutes.* A holder should be used to remove the hot test tube from the cup to protect the fingers, and the test tube should be placed in the small glass.

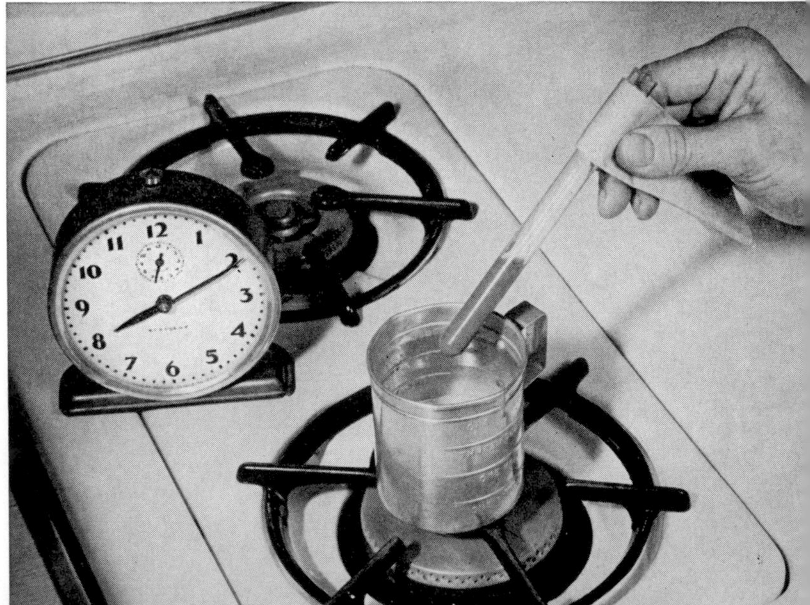

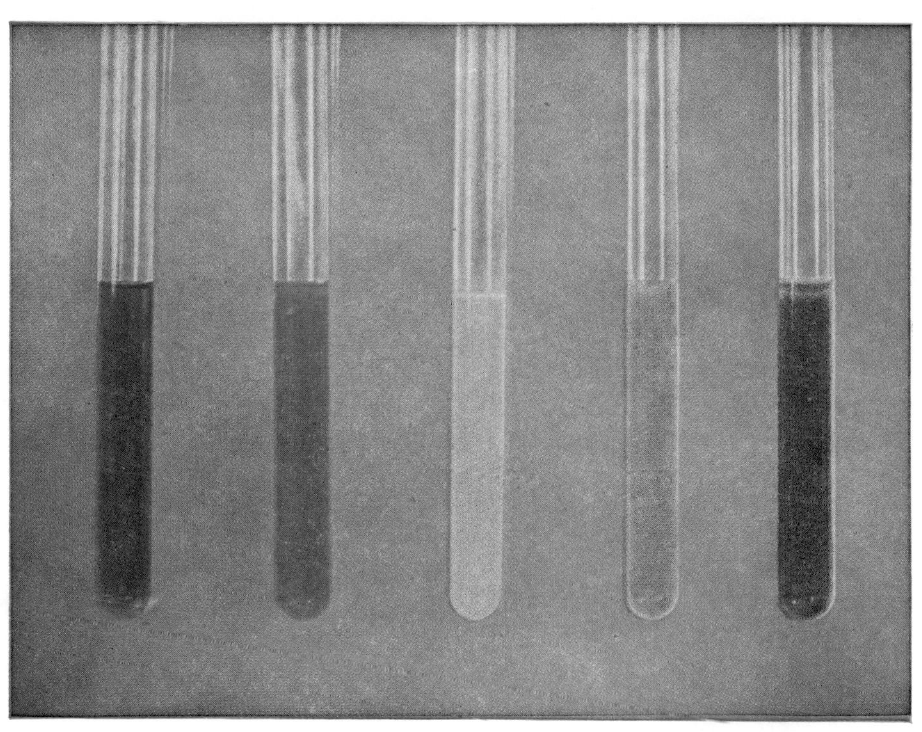

No sugar — Trace of sugar — (About) 1% sugar — More than 1% sugar — More than 2% sugar

PLATE 6. *The color of the solution in the test tube shows the amount of sugar in the urine.*

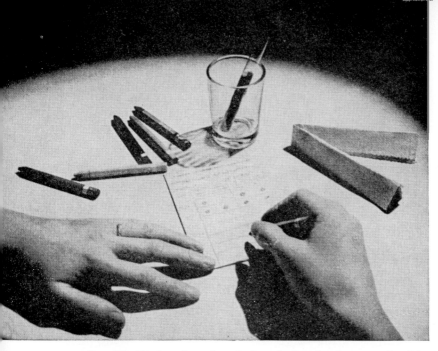

Fig. 71. *Notice the color of the solution in the test tube.* The color may be recorded with crayons on a special chart.

Fig. 72. Wash the articles on the tray after completing the test so that they may be ready for the next test. The stopper is placed back on the bottle of Benedict's solution. The cup, the container for urine and the small glass to hold the test tube are turned upside down on the tray.

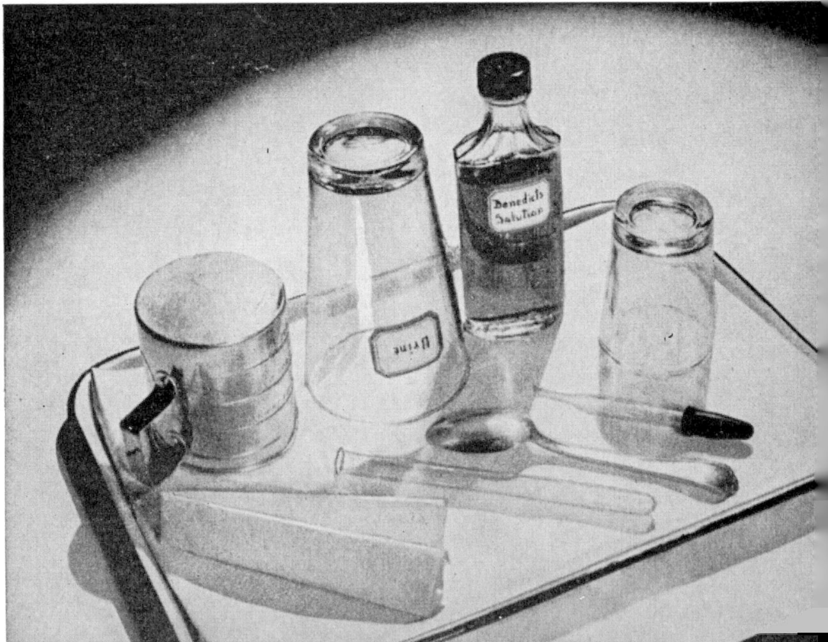

TEST FOR SUGAR IN THE URINE

CLINITEST*

(Urine Sugar Analysis Test)

PREPARATION

1. *A tray set up with the necessary equipment* is a convenience to the patient. The articles necessary for the test for sugar in the urine are: Clinitest Set, which contains Clinitest Tablets, a test tube, a medicine dropper and a color scale showing the amounts of sugar in the urine; a container for collecting the specimen of urine and a container for water (a small glass or a paper cup may be used) (Fig. 73).

PROCEDURE

2. *Open up Clinitest Set and place bottle of Clinitest Tablets on the tray* (Fig. 74).

3. *Always make certain that the Clinitest Tablet has a spotted bluish-white color.* Never use a tablet that has turned dark blue or any other color than bluish-white.

4. *Fill the medicine dropper with water* (Fig. 75).

5. *Place 10 drops of water in the test tube* (Fig. 76).

6. *Fill the medicine dropper with urine* (Fig. 77).

7. *Add 5 drops of urine to the water in the test tube* (Fig. 78).

8. *Remove 1 Clinitest Tablet from the bottle* (Fig. 79).

9. *Return the bottle cap immediately* (Fig. 80).

10. *Drop 1 Clinitest Tablet into the test tube containing the water and the urine.* Watch but do not touch the test tube while the reaction is taking place (Fig. 81).

11. *Wait for 15 seconds after the boiling inside the test tube has stopped, then lift the test tube from its holder and shake it gently* (Fig. 82).

12. *The color of the solution in the test tube shows the amount of sugar in the urine.* Compare solution in test tube with color scale (Plate 7).

13. *Record with crayon the color of the solution in the test tube.* Use the appropriate column of the Urine Analysis Record provided in the Clinitest Set or by your physician (Fig. 83).

14. *Wash the test tube, the medicine dropper and the containers for water and urine, so that they may be ready for the next test* (Fig. 84).

* Ames Company, Inc. Elkhart, Ind.

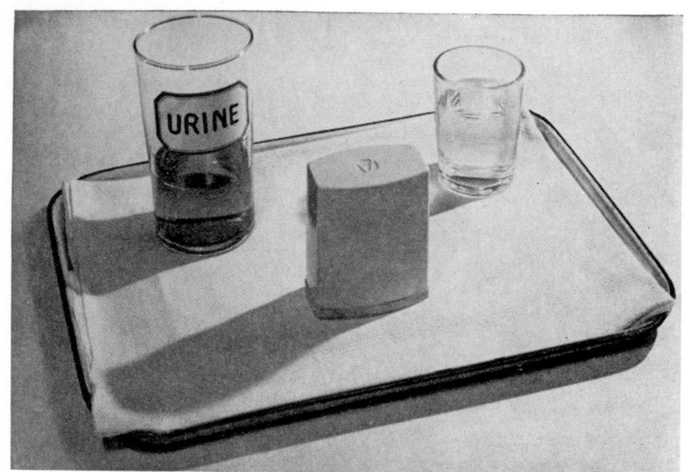

Fig. 73. *A tray set up with the necessary equipment* is a convenience to the patient. The articles necessary for the test for sugar in the urine are: Clinitest Set, which contains Clinitest Tablets, test tube, medicine dropper and color scale showing the amounts of sugar in the urine; container for collecting specimen of urine and container for water (small glass or paper cup may be used).

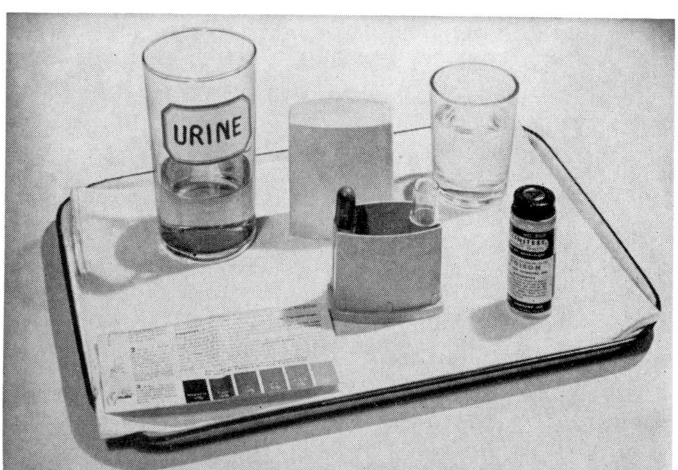

Fig. 74. *Open up Clinitest Set and place bottle of Clinitest Tablets on the tray.*

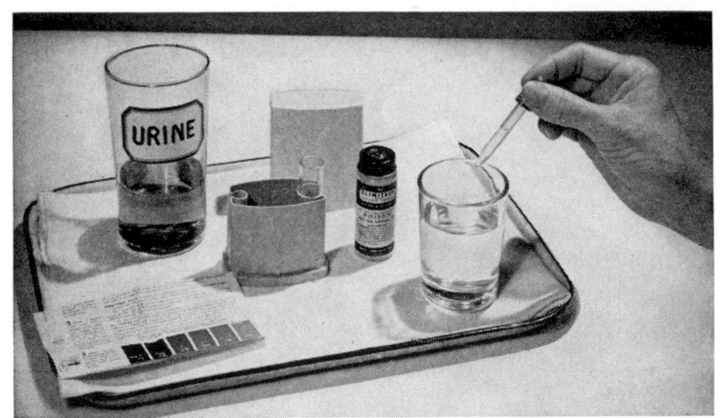

Fig. 75. *Fill the medicine dropper with water.*

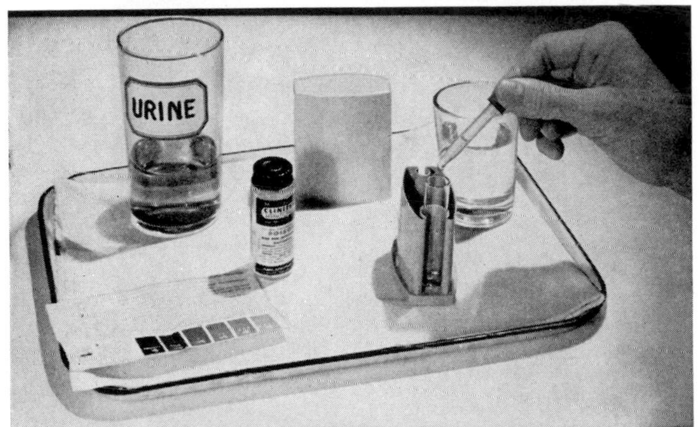

Fig. 76. *Place 10 drops of water in the test tube.*

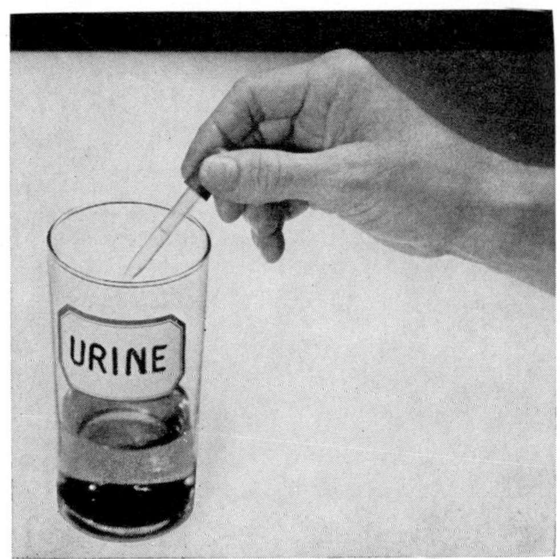

Fig. 77. *Fill the medicine dropper with urine.*

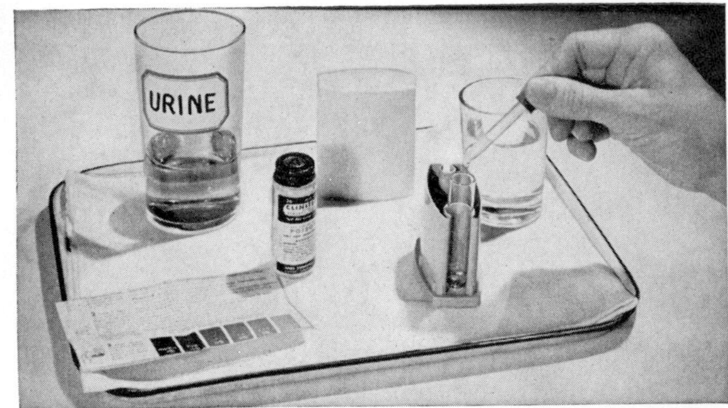

Fɪɢ. 78. *Add 5 drops of urine to the water in the test tube.*

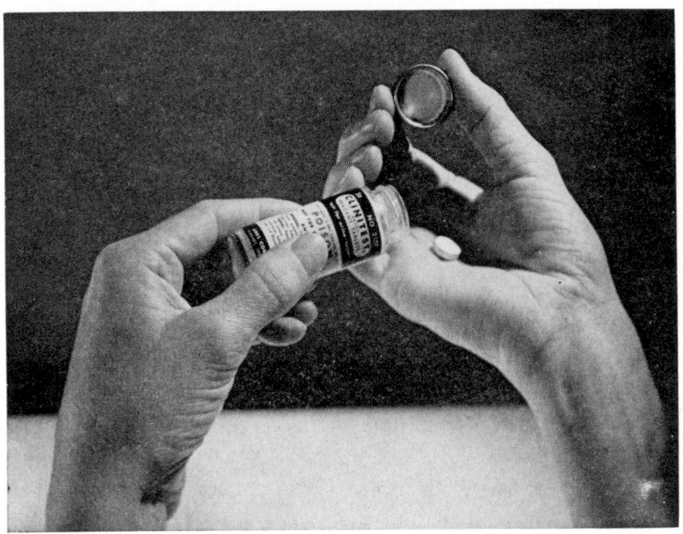

Fɪɢ. 79. *Remove 1 Clinitest Tablet from the bottle. Always make certain that the Clinitest Tablet has a spotted bluish-white color.* Never use a tablet that has turned dark blue or is any color other than bluish-white.

Fɪɢ. 80. *Return the bottle cap immediately.*

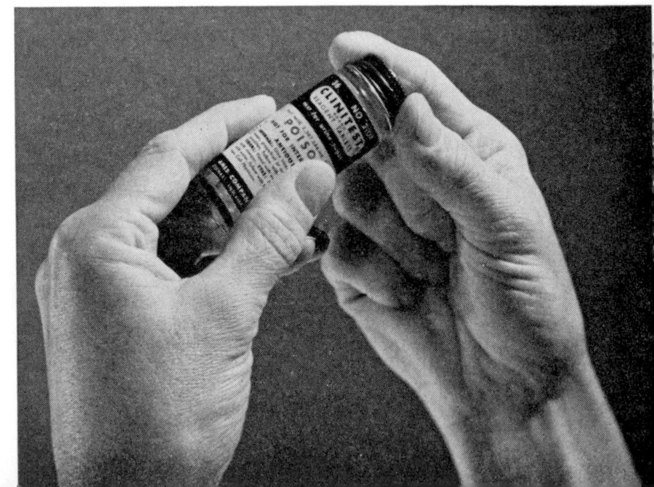

Fig. 81. *Drop 1 Clinitest Tablet into the test tube containing the water and the urine.* Watch but do not touch the test tube while the reaction is taking place.

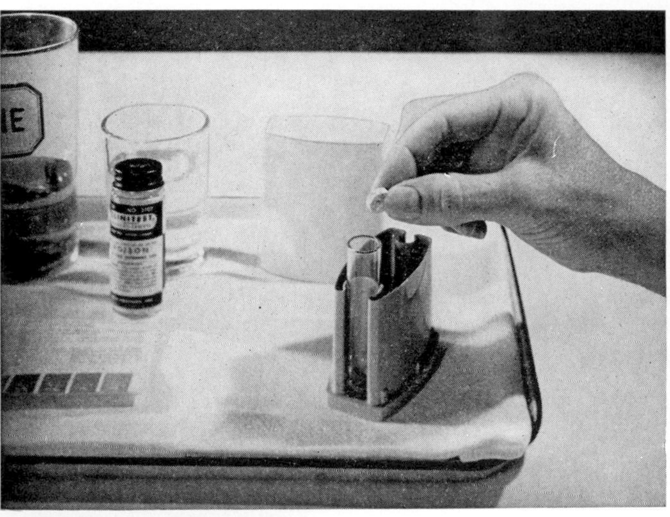

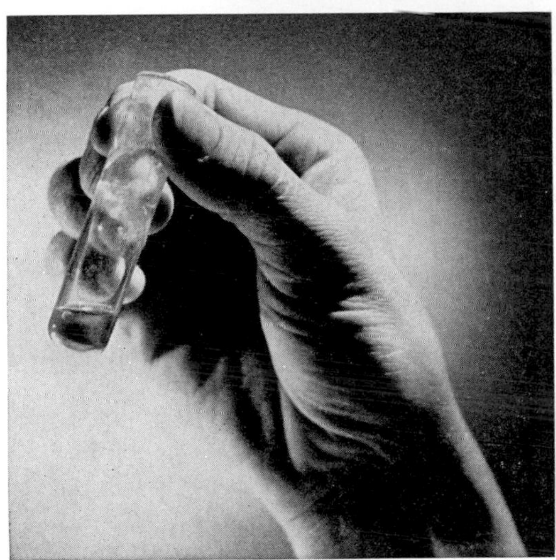

Fig. 82. *Wait for 15 seconds after the boiling inside the test tube has stopped, then lift the test tube from its holder and shake it gently.*

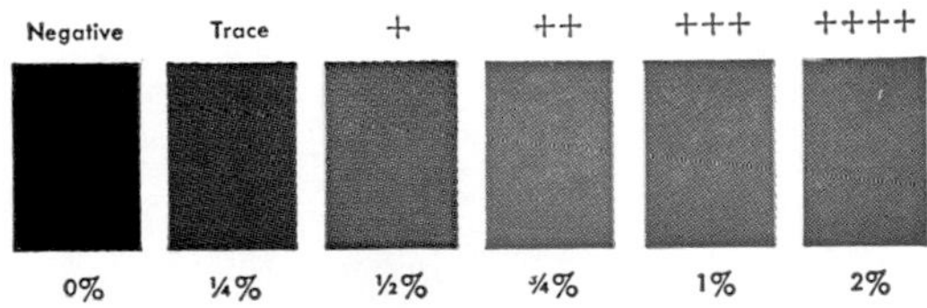

Plate 7. *The color of the solution in the test tube shows the amount of sugar in the urine.* Compare solution in test tube with color scale. (Ames Co., Elkhart, Ind.)

Fig. 83. *Record with crayon the color of the solution in the test tube.* Use the appropriate column of the Urine Analysis Record provided in the Clinitest Set or by your physician.

Fig. 84. *Wash the test tube, the medicine dropper and the containers for water and urine, so that they may be ready for the next test.*

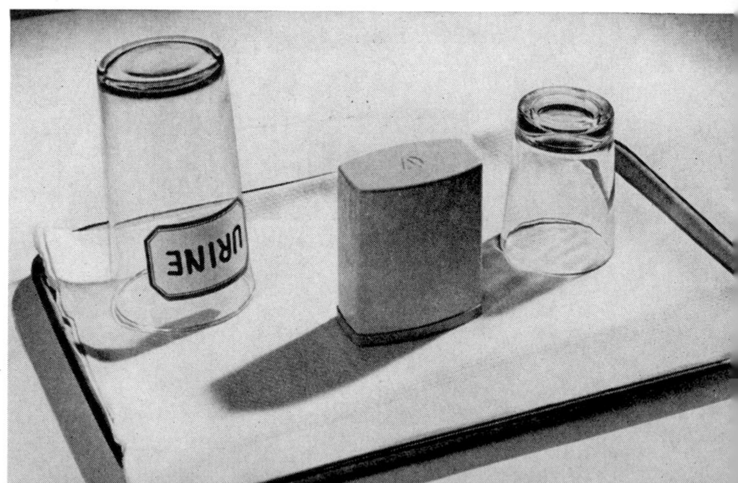

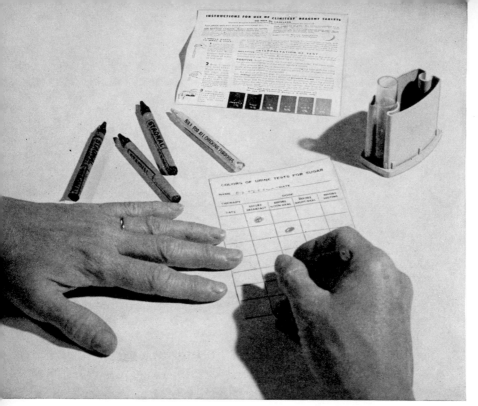

TEST FOR SUGAR IN THE URINE

TES-TAPE

(Urine Sugar Analysis Paper)

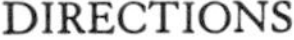
DIRECTIONS

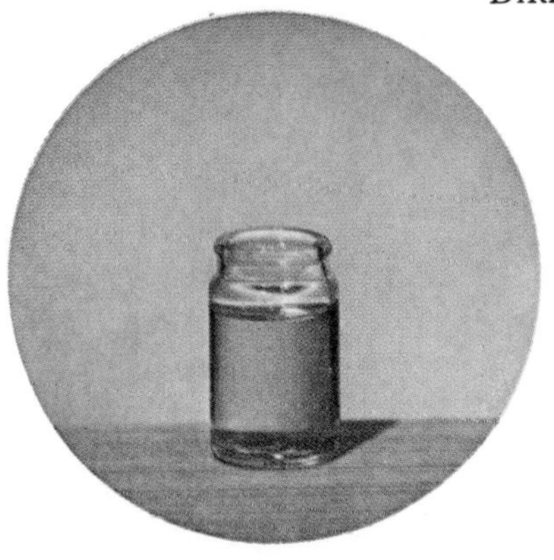

1. Collect urine specimen.

Special equipment is not required for the collection of urine. Be careful to avoid use of a container contaminated with sugar (glucose).

Withdraw about 1½ inches of 'Tes-Tape' by pulling down, and tear by pulling up against the cutting edge.

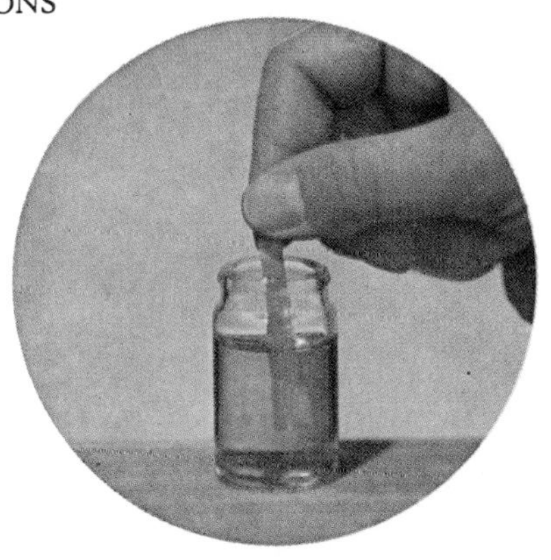

2. Moisten the strip of 'Tes-Tape' with urine.

The quantity of urine needed is very small. Uniform moistening of strip will assure the most accurate indication. Since the hands may carry traces of sugar, the end of the tape held between the fingers should be kept dry.

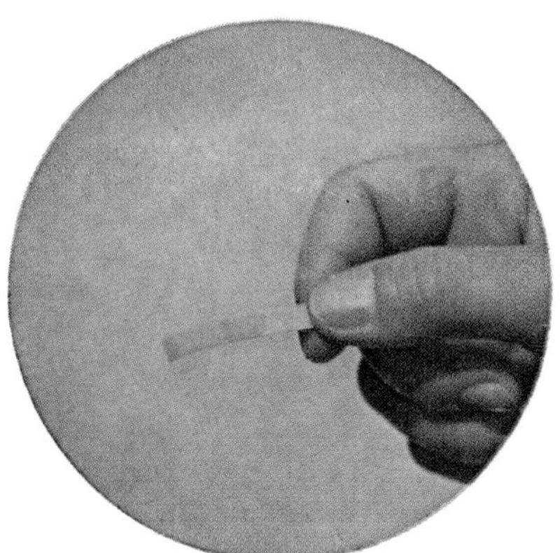

3. Wait for one minute.

Calibrated color development in the moistened tape is accomplished in one minute. During this time, the tape should be held as pictured. (Laying the tape on a dish, paper, or other surface may result in a false reading because of sugar contamination.) *Yellow color indicates urine is sugar-free.*

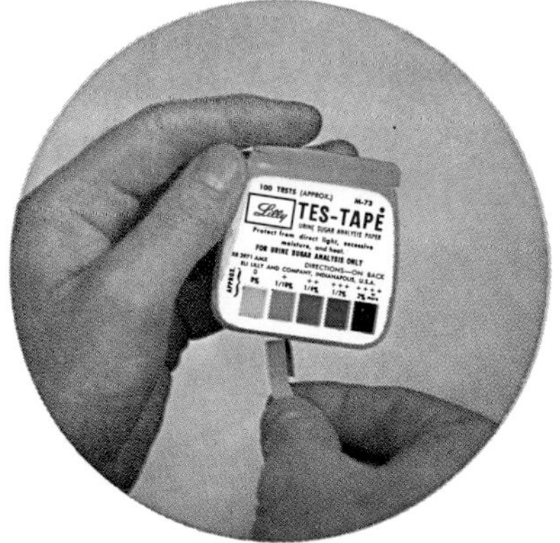

4. Then *immediately* compare darkest area on tape with the color chart on the dispenser.

If tape indicates ½ percent or higher, wait one additional minute and make final comparison. When the 'Tes-Tape' strip is matched with the color chart, the reading indicates the amount of glucose either in percent or in relative figures (0 to ++++).

PLATE 8 (Eli Lilly and Company, Indianapolis, Ind.)

TEST FOR SUGAR IN THE URINE

CLINISTIX*

DIRECTIONS FOR TEST †

1. Dip test area (red-colored end) of strip in fresh, well mixed urine, or pass test area of strip through urine stream. Remove immediately.

2. Compare color of test area with color chart, 10 (ten) *seconds* after wetting.

INTERPRETATION OF TEST

Negative: No purple color. Test area remains red.

Positive: Purple color present in test area.

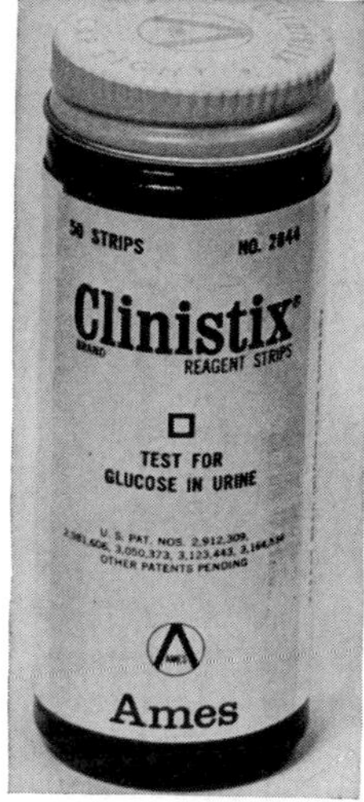

FIGURE 85

---

* Ames Company.

† Directions are enclosed in each Clinistix package and on the label on the bottle. They should be read carefully.

URINE TEST FOR ACETONE (KETONES)
ACETEST*

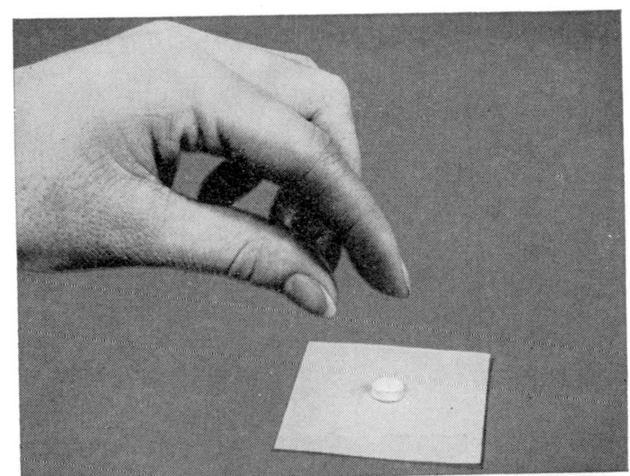

THREE SIMPLE STEPS FOR USE OF ACETEST

1. Place the Acetest tablet on a clean surface, preferably a piece of paper.

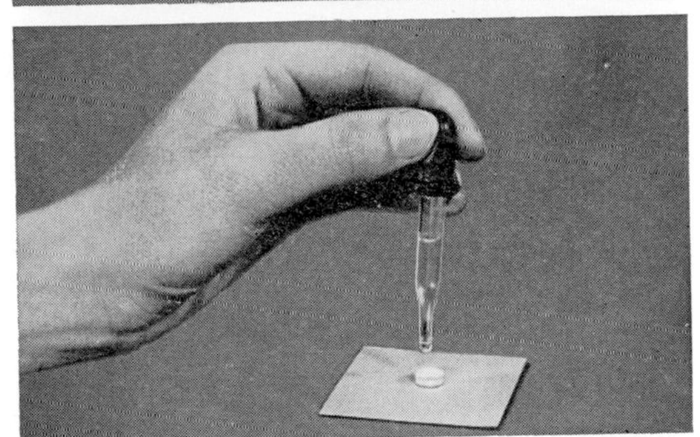

2. Put *one* drop of urine on the tablet.

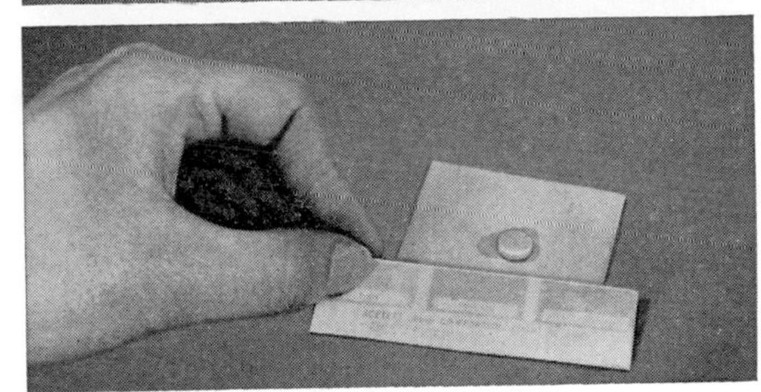

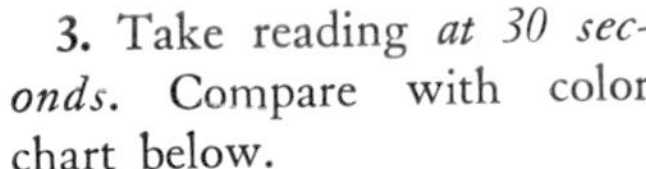

3. Take reading *at 30 seconds.* Compare with color chart below.

INTERPRETATION OF TEST

Negative: Tablet color will remain unchanged or turn cream-colored from wetting.

Positive: Within 30 seconds, color of tablet will change. Depending on amount of Ketone bodies present, color varies from lavender to deep purple. Results may be recorded as small, moderate or large amount.

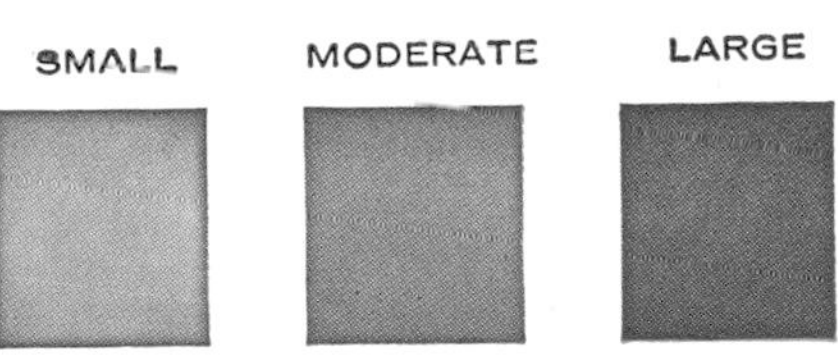

PLATE 9

* Ames Co., Inc., Elkhart, Ind.

URINE TEST FOR ACETONE (KETONES)
KETOSTIX*

DIRECTIONS FOR TEST†

1. Dip test area (yellow-colored end) of strip briefly into fresh, well-mixed urine or pass test area of strip through urine stream.

2. Compare color of test area with color chart 15 (fifteen) *seconds* after wetting.

INTERPRETATION OF TEST

Negative: No purple color develops. Test area remains yellow.

Positive: Purple color develops in test area.

---

* Ames Company.

† Directions are written on the inside of the carton containing bottle of reagent strips. They should be read carefully.

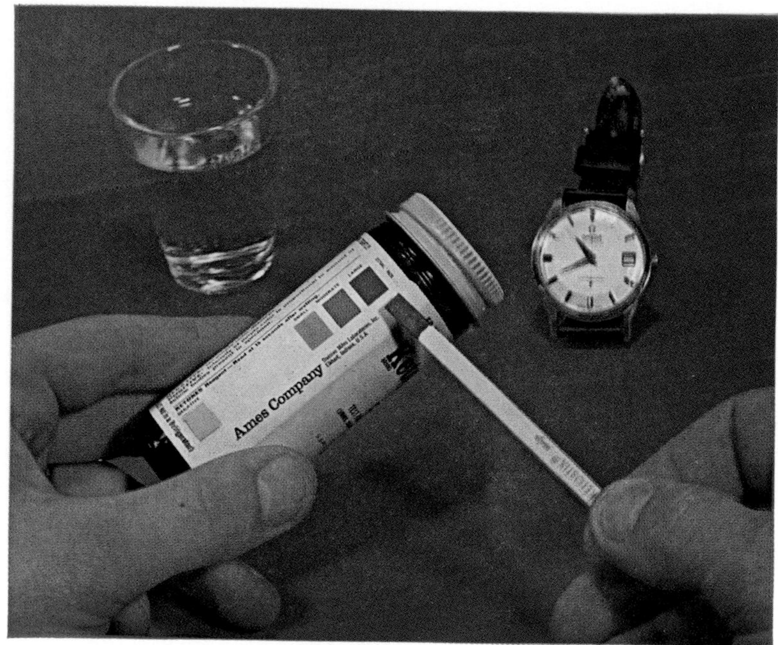

PLATE 10

7. SKIN INJURIES AND INFECTIONS FROM SKIN INJURIES

DIABETES AND INFECTIONS

The Skin is a protective covering for the body, and while it remains unbroken infection from without will rarely occur. Any injury to the skin, no matter how slight, should be given immediate care to guard against possible infections. Infections are especially serious, as they often cause diabetes to become temporarily more severe. Often, during the period of infection, the dosage of insulin may need to be increased. Frequently, during this time, a patient who has been controlled with diet alone, or with diet and an oral agent may require insulin. When diabetes is uncontrolled it is believed that infections are more likely to develop, and when infections are present with uncontrolled diabetes there is danger of acidosis.

Any damage to the skin, whether slight or severe, must be considered as an injury. Slight injuries are scratches, scrapes, small cuts, broken or cracked skin (fissures) and hangnails. The more severe conditions are ulcers, boils (furuncles), carbuncles, abscesses, blisters, deep cuts, burns, sunburn and complications which result from overexposure to cold.

PREVENTION OF SKIN INJURIES

Often skin injuries can be prevented. Breaks or cracks in the skin may be the result of dry skin, in which case they can be prevented by applying lanolin to keep the skin soft and smooth. However, when cracks or breaks in the skin occur between the toes, lanolin should not be used, as these commonly indicate a fungus infection (athlete's foot) and require medical care. Blisters caused by friction can be prevented by careful selection of shoes and stockings (see Chap. 8). Burns caused by overexposure to the sun or sun lamps are serious and should be prevented by gradual exposure. There are special lotions for protection. Precautions should also be taken when using lamps, heating pads and hot-water bottles. Injuries caused by frostbite or overexposure to cold carry great risk of serious damage to the skin and the underlying tissues and can be avoided by protecting the body with sufficiently warm clothing. Hand injuries often result from the use of common household cleaning fluids, powders and disinfectants, many of which are irritating and injurious to the skin and should not be used unless the hands are protected. The hands should also be protected when any cleaning materials that might damage the skin are being used, for example, metallic sponges, scouring pads or other types of abrasives may produce breaks in the skin and open a path for infection.

TREATMENT OF SKIN INJURIES

Prompt care of skin injuries, no matter how slight, is essential in preventing the development or the spread of infections and harm to the deeper tissues. A physician should treat severe injuries, as well as slight injuries that do not heal readily.

The simplest and safest way to treat slight injuries is to bathe the affected part with mild soap and warm water, wiping it with cotton that has been dipped in alcohol and then applying a sterile gauze pad or dressing.* Such dressings can be purchased in individual packages and always should be kept available. The hands should be washed before touching the sterile dressing, and the surface of the dressing to be applied to the injured area should not be touched by the hands or any object. Bandages that are used to hold the dressing in place must be clean and should not be wrapped tightly, as they may interfere with circulation. Adhesive tape should be used sparingly, if at all, since it may irritate the skin or break it when the tape is being removed.

Only such antiseptics as have been prescribed by the physician should be used, since many common antiseptics may irritate, burn or further injure the skin. Antiseptics that should *not* be used in ointment or liquid form include the following: iodine, carbolic acid or phenol, bichloride of mercury, oil of mustard, cantharidin, salicylic acid and Capsicum. The names of these substances, which usually do not appear in the trade name of the product, are printed on the label where the contents or the ingredients are stated. The label on the container should be read carefully before any antiseptic is used.

With the advent in recent years of chemical agents and antibiotics, most infections can now be treated successfully, and surgery in the presence of infection no longer carries as great a risk. Many lives have been saved as a result of these newer therapeutic agents.

* Soaps containing antibacterial agents such as hexachlorophene may be used.

8. PERSONAL HYGIENE, EXERCISE AND SPECIAL CARE OF CERTAIN PARTS OF THE BODY

PERSONAL HYGIENE

HYGIENE, being the art of health preservation, whether physical or mental, is advocated as a regular practice for everyone. There can be no question that good habits or high hygienic standards are essential to the good health of all. Hygiene assumes even greater importance when diabetes is present, because its control depends to a great extent upon the establishment of regularity in everyday activities. It is especially important that the person who takes insulin realize this and plan a daily routine which allows sufficient time for meals, exercise, sleep, rest and recreation. The patient with controlled diabetes usually can engage in most activities or occupations provided that a regular routine is followed and assuming that there is no other condition to warrant restrictions. It is well to remember that worry and anxiety may have an unfavorable effect on the diabetes which is often evidenced by increased amounts of sugar in the blood and in the urine.

Cleanliness of the body, and especially of the feet (p. 177), the teeth, the hands and the nails, is important, not only for the prevention of infections (Chap. 7) but also for desirable daily living conditions. There should be sufficient conveniences in the home, the school, the place of occupation and the community to meet the needs for good sanitation, as well as for the prevention of communicable diseases.

Sleep and Rest. An adequate amount of sleep and rest is essential, since the strain of overfatigue may be upsetting. Sleeping conditions should provide restful sleep—comfortable beds, proper temperature and ventilation. Sleeping quarters should be so arranged that the patient who may wish to rest during the day or to retire early can do so without being disturbed. Fatigue from overactivity or lack of proper rest may affect the appetite so unfavorably that the patient does not take the amount of food that has been prescribed.

Bowel Elimination. Good habits of bowel elimination depend not only on the kinds and the amounts of food and fluid that are taken in but also on the daily routine and the toilet facilities in the home, the school or the place of occupation. It is essential to establish good habits of bowel elimination. This means allowing sufficient time at a definite period in the day's routine.

Exercise is an important component of diabetic treatment. In addition to the promotion of physical fitness, exercise also enhances the utilization of sugar, often diminishes the required amount of insulin and is particularly valuable in improving and stimulating the circulation in the body.

Unless contraindicated for other physical reasons, a moderate amount of daily exercise is desirable. The type, the amount and the frequency should be planned with the guidance of the physician. Once decided, there should be concerted effort to follow the same regimen each day so that unnecessary fluctuations in blood-sugar levels will be minimized or avoided. Regular planned activity is especially important when treatment includes insulin or oral drug therapy.

There may be times when there are variations in the daily activity. There are ways to compensate for these variations. When more than the usual amount of exercise is planned, the diet may need to be increased. Extra carbohydrate in the form of fruit or fruit juice often is recommended before short periods of exercise, while longer periods of exercise require, in addition to the fruit, other foods that contain all 3 food constituents—carbohydrate, protein and fat. Foods such as milk, bread and butter or their food exchanges are recommended. These will furnish additional sugar for energy requirements for a longer period of time. Carbohydrate, which can be used by the body quickly and is readily available as a source of sugar, should be kept handy in the event of an insulin reaction. This could include such foods as sugar, candy, fruit, fruit juice or soft drinks (tonic or pop).

When the usual daily amount of physical activity is decreased, the diet frequently needs to be lessened. When food adjustments are not effective for this purpose, there may be need for the adjustment of the dosage of insulin or oral agent. This manipulation is not usually recommended when dietary adjustment is effective and satisfactory.

Many patients may find that urine-sugar is increased during weekends even though the diabetes is well controlled during the weekdays. This weekend situation can be remedied either by a small reduction in diet, an increase in activity, or by a slight increase in the dosage of insulin or oral agent. Any deviation from the prescribed treatment must not be attempted by the patient. Adjustments are made by the physician.

THE EYES

A yearly examination by an eye specialist is important, as changes in vision are often associated with diabetes. There may be temporary variations in the acuity of vision which results from fluctuations or prolonged elevations of blood-sugar levels. This condition often occurs when treatment is first instituted or when the diabetes is uncontrolled and becomes stabilized when the diabetes becomes controlled. It is usually advisable not to have glasses fitted or changed until good control is attained.

More important and serious are the changes that may take place in the retina (the sensitive membrane of the eye). This condition, called retinitis, often results in a diminution of vision in varying degrees and may be difficult to correct. However, especially good and persistent control of the diabetes may help to allay the onset of this condition and to slow the progress. Cataracts (opacities in the lens of the eye) sometimes develop and may interfere with vision. However, when mature, these usually can be removed surgically to achieve restoration of vision.

THE TEETH

Regular visits to the dentist are desirable to maintain good repair of the teeth. When dentures are worn, the mouth should be examined at regular intervals to make certain that they fit properly and are not causing gum irritation. Any tooth or gum infection requires immediate treatment. The dentist should always be informed of the diabetic condition.

When extractions are necessary it is well, if possible, to choose a time when the diabetes is controlled. The number of teeth to be extracted at one time should be decided by both the physician and the dentist.

When the gums are sore or tender the food in the prescribed diet should be so prepared that chewing is made easy or even unnecessary. Fruits and vegetables can be used in the form of juices or can be cooked and mashed, and meat and poultry can be ground. The other foods in the diet usually do not require special preparation (pp. 78, 80 and 82).

THE HAIR

A haircut, a shave or removal of hair in any way should be done with care to prevent skin infections caused by ingrowing hairs or the use of razors, scissors, clippers or other equipment that is not clean. Ingrowing hairs often result from shaving too closely or from the use of depilatories (hair removers). The hair on the neck should be removed with a clipper or scissors (not shaved), and depilatories should be used with caution.

THE HANDS

The hands come in contact with many objects and often are carriers of infection. Mild soap and warm water should be used when washing the hands. Care should be taken to dry the hands thoroughly to avoid chapping. Fingernails should be kept at the proper length. The cuticle may be pushed back gently with an orange-wood stick but never with a pointed or sharp instrument. Hangnails and injuries to the skin round the nails should be cared for at once (Chap. 7) to prevent infection.

THE FEET

The proper care of the feet is of extreme importance to prevent the development of serious conditions. More than any other part of the body, the feet are affected by the condition of the circulation. The blood flows through blood vessels which are shaped like tubes. The space inside the wall of the blood vessel is called the lumen. When circulation is good the blood-vessel walls are soft and elastic, so that the blood flows through them with ease. However, as a person grows older certain changes take place in the blood vessels. The walls become thicker and harder, and the elasticity is lessened. The lumen, through which the blood flows, becomes narrower, which results in decreased blood flow (Fig. 86).

In the presence of impaired circulation one or more of the following conditions may occur. Often there is a burning feeling, or the feet may be cold, numb, or even painful at times. Walking may cause a tired feeling or cramps in the toes, the feet or the legs. Any unusual condition of the feet, such as swelling, pain, soreness and changes in the color of the skin, should be reported to the physician.

When there is evidence of impairment of circulation *the use of tobacco is usually prohibited. Rest periods are often recommended,* during which time the legs should be elevated. *Massaging the feet and the legs* may be helpful. This is done by spreading lanolin on the hands and kneading the flesh gently from the toes to the knees. *Warm baths or whirlpool baths may be beneficial for some patients. Warm stockings and storm boots should be worn during cold weather. Woolen bedsocks may be used at night,* but hot-water bags, electric heating pads or other heating appliances should be used only to warm the bed and should not be placed on the feet at any time, since they may cause a burn. *Crossing the knees or sitting on the legs interferes with circulation.* The legs should be crossed at the ankles only.

Any special treatment for impaired circulation is prescribed by the physician. *Contrast baths,* which are recommended occasionally, consist of placing the feet and the lower part of the legs, immediately above the ankles, first in warm water (105° F.) for 1 minute or longer, as directed, and then for the same length of time in cold water (50° F.). Always begin and end with warm water. It is wise to use a bath thermometer to obtain the correct tem-

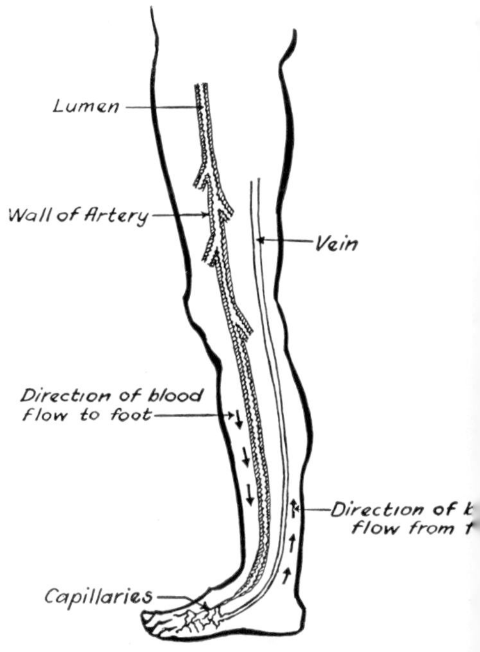

Fig. 86. Diagram of the circulation in the foot and the leg.

perature. However, if a thermometer is not available, the water should be tested with the elbow or the wrist.

The Buerger-Allen exercise is commonly recommended in an attempt to improve circulation. Figures 87 to 92 show the procedure for the various parts of this exercise. The physician will prescribe the number of times this exercise is to be repeated.

BUERGER-ALLEN EXERCISE

The exercise, consisting of 3 parts, should be repeated as many times as the physician prescribes.

Part I

Lie down on a bed or a couch and elevate both feet on a Buerger's Board (Fig. 87) from ½ to 3 minutes. A straight-backed chair (Fig. 88) may be used instead to elevate the feet by resting the top of the back of it and the front of the seat on the bed or the couch. Place a soft covering or a pillow on the back of the chair or the board.

Figure 87

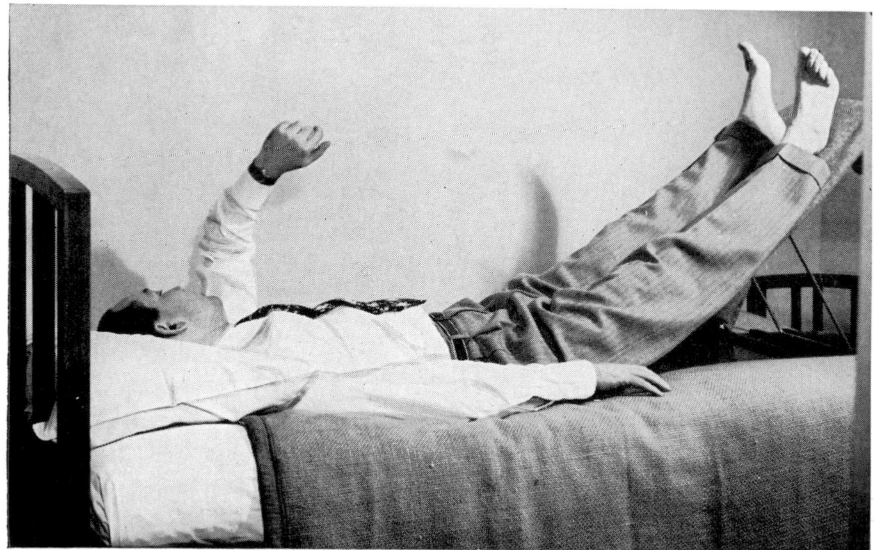

Figure 88

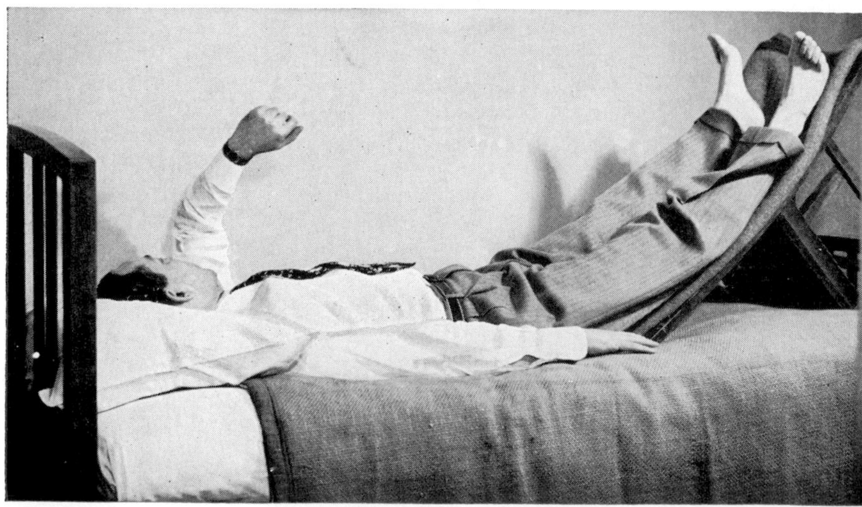

SHOES AND STOCKINGS

Special care is necessary in the selection of shoes. Each part of the shoe must be considered for the protection it gives to every part of the foot when at rest or used in standing, walking, running or for other activities (Fig. 93). The shoes should always allow the feet to rest in their natural position for freedom of movement, support of body weight and good posture (Fig. 94).

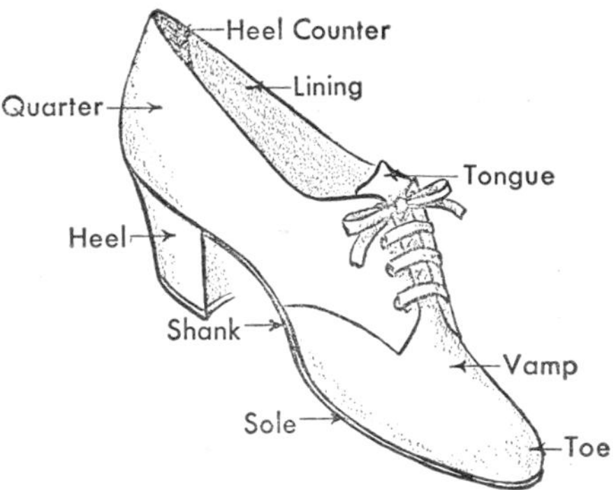

Fig. 93. The parts of the shoe.

Selection of Shoes

Size of shoes

Length. Measure foot from the back of the heel to the tip of the big toe. Shoe should extend ¾ of an inch beyond the big toe when standing. The length from the back of the heel to the ball of the foot should also be known to ensure correct fit

Width. Measure across the ball of the foot

Parts of the shoe (Fig. 93)

Upper Part. Of soft leather

Outer Line of Sole. Should fit the natural curve of the outer side of the foot

Inside Line of Sole. Straight, or nearly so, to allow room for the big toe to move forward when standing or walking

Toe. Round and high with plenty of room for toes to move freely

Vamp. Should support the foot, yet give it plenty of room

Sole. Made of leather that can be bent easily. Rubber may be placed on leather soles, but wooden soles should not be used

Tongue. Should have no rough seams that might hurt the foot and should be wide enough to protect the feet from ridges caused by lacings and eyelets

Shank. Stiff and as wide as the arch of the foot

Lining. Smooth, with no wrinkles or rough edges that might irritate the foot

Heel. Broad at the base. Heels of women's shoes should be no more than 1¼inches in height

Quarter. Should fit the heel and the arch of the foot snugly so that the foot is kept in its natural position in the shoe

Heel Counter. Firm, but soft enough

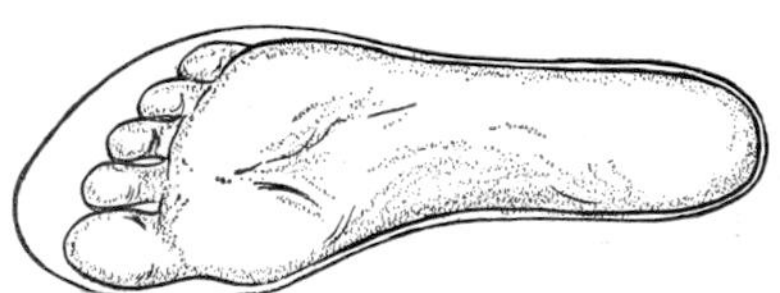

Fig. 94. The natural position of the foot in the shoe.

so that the foot will not be irritated

New shoes usually should be worn at first only for a short period of time. It is well to have an extra pair of shoes so that the same pair is not worn every day. Shoes should be kept in good repair, especially the heels, and old shoes that do not support the feet should not be worn. Shoe lacings should not be tied so tightly as to interfere with circulation. Eyelets should be smooth to avoid irritation. It is well to use a shoehorn so that the heel counter may be kept firm. House slippers should be chosen with the same care as shoes for the support and the protection of the feet. Bedroom slippers should be used only as a covering for bare feet when getting out of bed.

Selection of Stockings

Stockings

Size. One half inch longer than the length of the foot

Dye. Fast colors, so that feet are not stained

Seams. Smooth, so that they do not cause irritation

Material. Not bulky, so that space allowed for the feet is not lessened. Woolen stockings absorb moisture and should be worn when feet perspire freely. They also are desirable for keeping the feet warm

When putting on stockings, they should be drawn carefully over the toes (Fig. 95). The toe of the stocking should be pulled out before putting on the shoe to leave plenty of room for the toes (Fig. 96). *Circular garters and rolled stockings can interfere with circulation and should not be worn.* Elasticized socks or stockings for both men and women should be chosen with care to make certain that there is no interference with circulation. New stockings should be washed before wearing. Stockings should be mended carefully so that there will be no rough places to cause irritation.

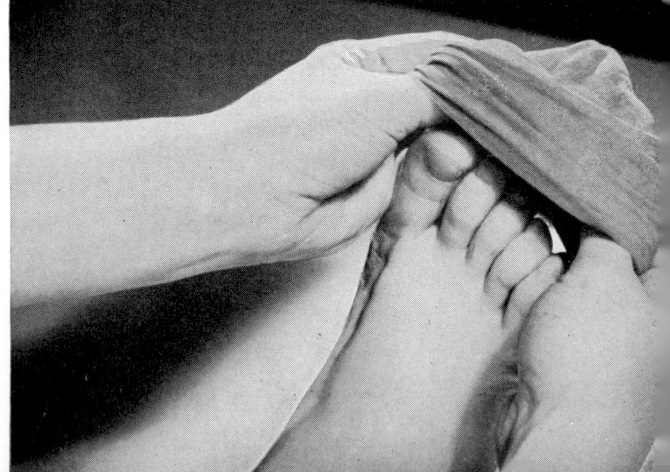

Fig. 95. When putting on stockings they should be drawn carefully over the toes.

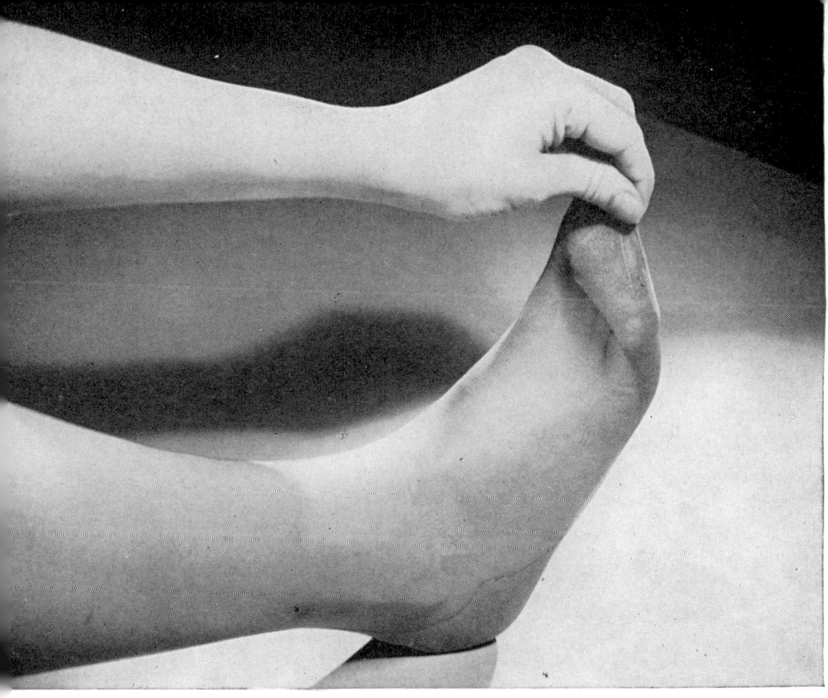

Fig. 96. The toe of the stocking should be pulled out before putting on the shoe to leave plenty of room.

BATHING THE FEET

Cleanliness of the body, and especially of the feet, is extremely important. The feet should be washed every day. The articles needed are a basin or a bathtub, a soft cloth, mild soap and warm (not hot) water (Fig. 97). The feet should be washed gently, and care should be taken not to break the skin between the toes (Fig. 98).

The feet should be dried with a smooth, soft towel (Fig. 99). Special care is necessary when drying the skin between the toes. The toes should be spread apart carefully, and the skin between them wiped gently until thoroughly dry. Then, dusting powder may be used, especially between the toes (Fig. 100).

When the feet are dry and scaly they should be wiped lightly with lanolin once a day but, to avoid collecting moisture, never between the toes (Fig. 101). The feet should not be allowed to become tender with too frequent use of lanolin. *When the feet perspire freely and are moist* they can be rubbed lightly with alcohol once or twice a day as necessary (Fig. 102).

The care of the toenails is an important part of the care of the feet. When the patient does not have good eyesight or steady hands someone else should care for his nails. Always in good light, the nails should be cut straight across and never cut shorter than the tips of the toes (Fig. 103). Sharp corners should be rounded and the nails cleaned with an orangewood stick, the tip wrapped with absorbent cotton (Fig. 104). In the same way, lanolin can be applied to the nails that are brittle and break easily—on the cuticle and under the nail (Fig. 105). Hangnails should be cut off as near the skin as possible.

Corns and Calluses. It is wise to have these treated by a chiropodist who has been informed of the presence of diabetes. Corns and calluses are the result of thickening of the skin, usually caused from the rubbing or pressure of shoes. The patient should never cut corns and calluses, for there is danger of injuring the skin and incurring infection. However, corns and calluses may be rubbed down carefully with a fine emery board after they have been well soaked. Corn remedies and corn cures should not be used. Corn pads should be used only on the advice of the physician or the chiropodist.

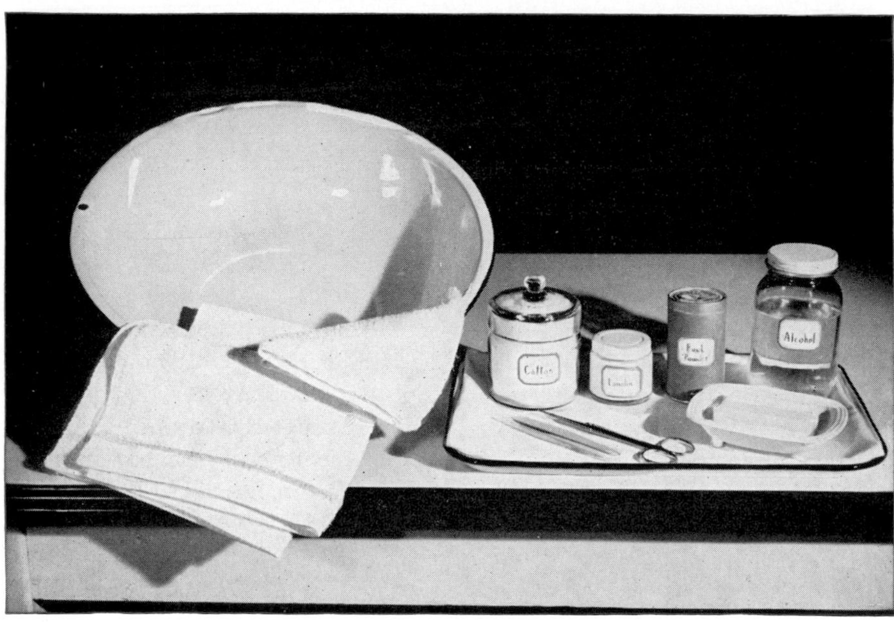

FIG. 97. The articles needed for the care of the feet are a basin or a bathtub, mild soap, such as may be used for the face, a soft washcloth and towel, warm (not hot) water, foot powder, lanolin, alcohol, absorbent cotton, an orangewood stick, an emery board and a pair of scissors (not pointed) or a large size nail clipper.

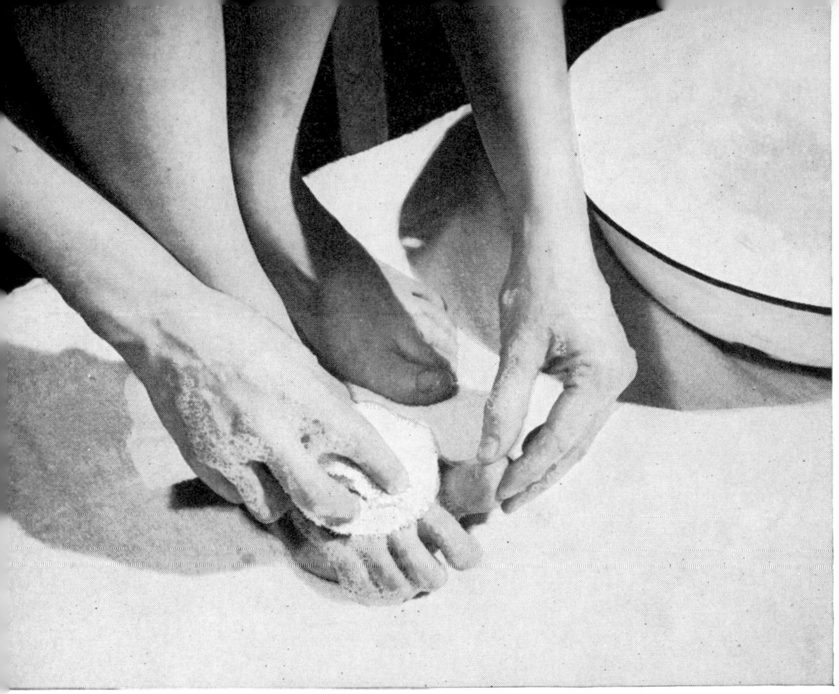

Fig. 98. The feet should be washed gently, and care should be taken not to break the skin between the toes.

Fig. 99. The feet should be dried with a smooth soft towel. Special care is necessary when drying the skin between the toes. The toes should be spread apart carefully, and the skin between them wiped gently until thoroughly dry.

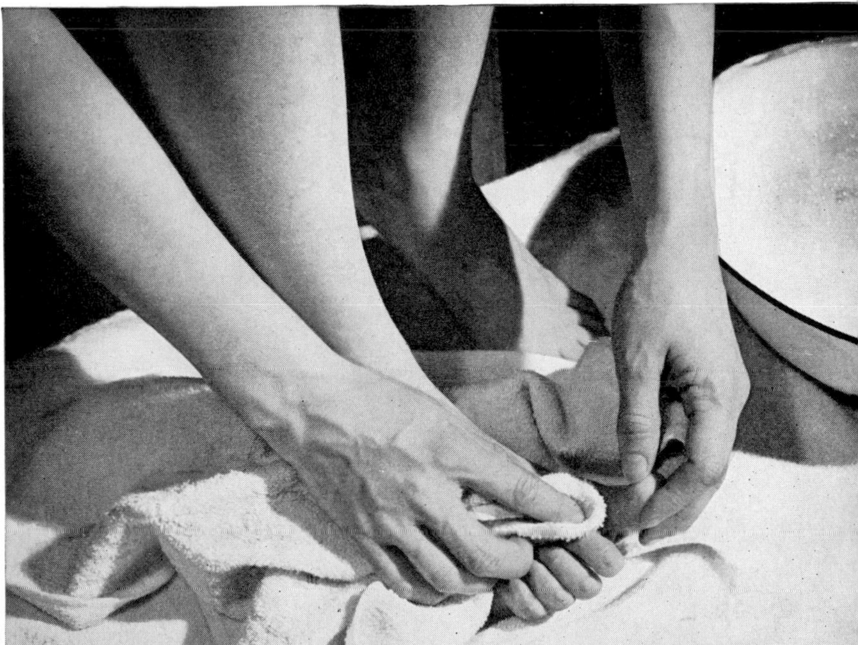

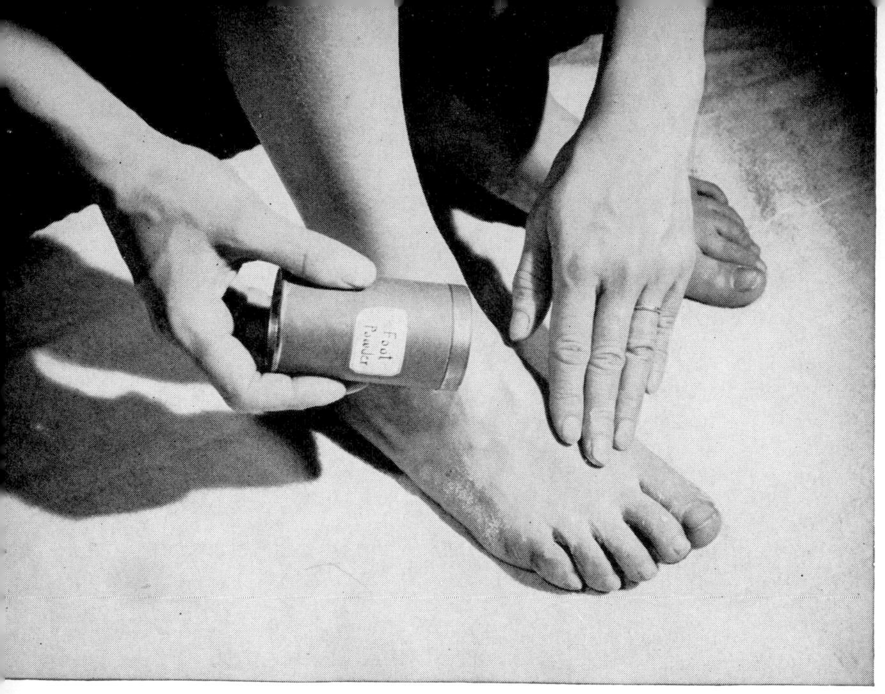

Fig. 100. Dusting powder may be used lightly, especially between the toes.

Fig. 101. When the feet are dry and scaly they should be wiped lightly with lanolin once a day but, to avoid collecting moisture, never between the toes. The feet should not be allowed to become tender with too frequent use of lanolin.

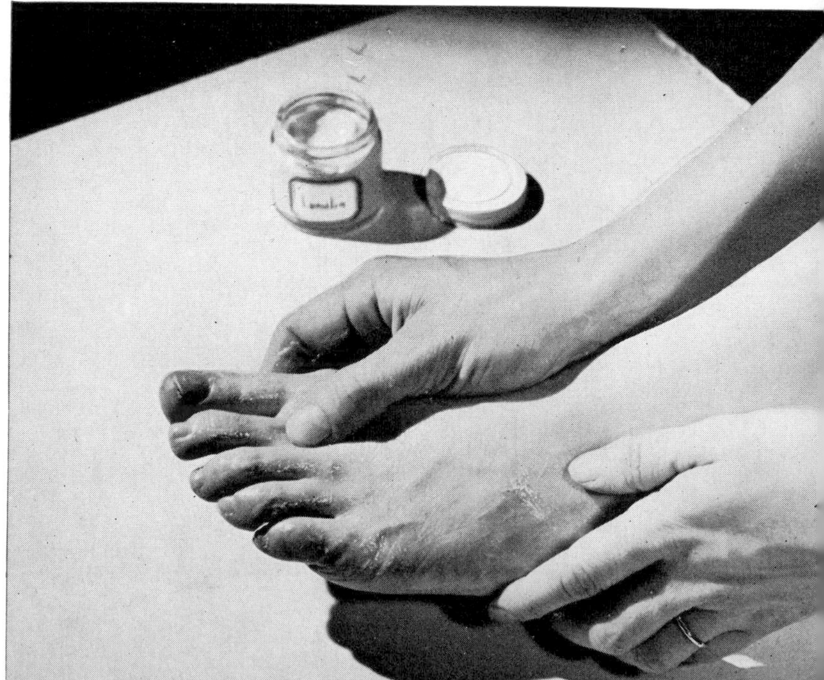

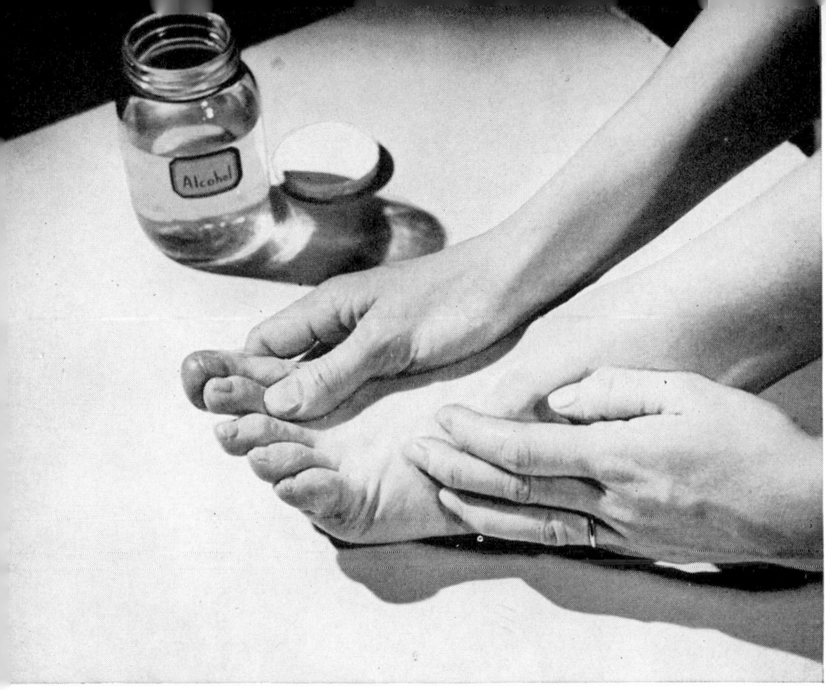

Fig. 102. When the feet perspire freely and are moist they can be stroked lightly with alcohol once or twice a day as necessary.

Fig. 103. The care of the toenails is an important part of the care of the feet. When the patient does not have good eyesight or steady hands someone else should care for his nails. Always in good light, nails should be cut straight across and never cut shorter than the tips of the toes. Sharp corners should be rounded.

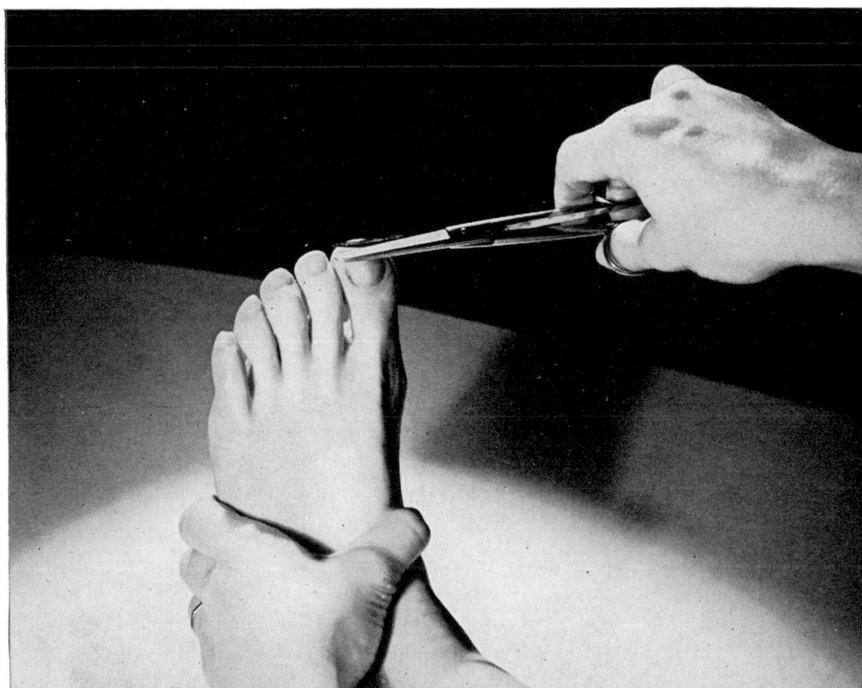

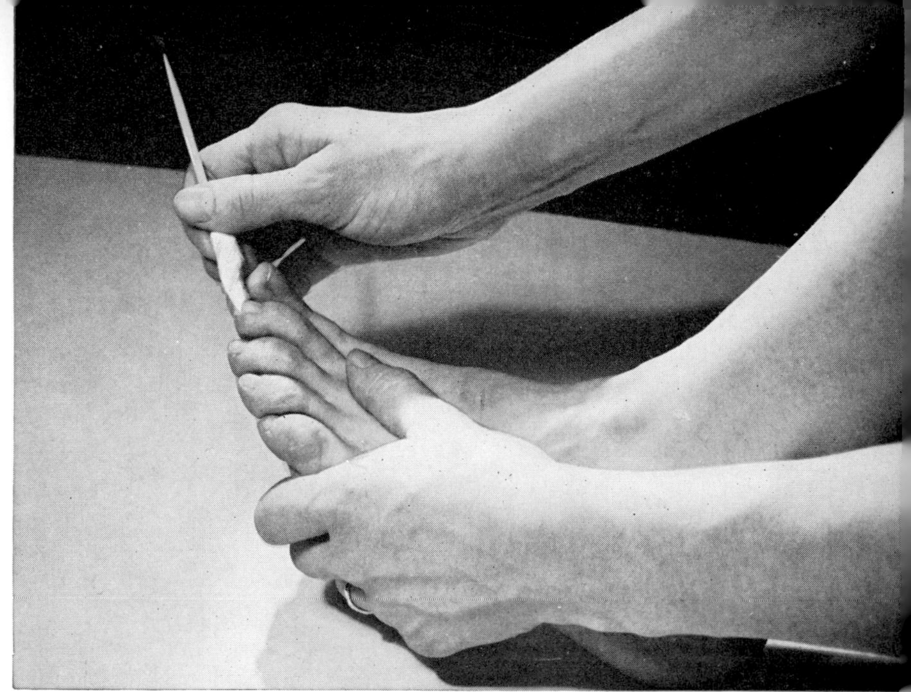

FIG. 104. Nails should be cleaned with an orangewood stick, the tip wrapped with absorbent cotton.

FIG. 105. Lanolin should be applied to nails that are brittle and break easily—on the cuticle and under the nail—with an orangewood stick that has been wrapped with absorbent cotton.

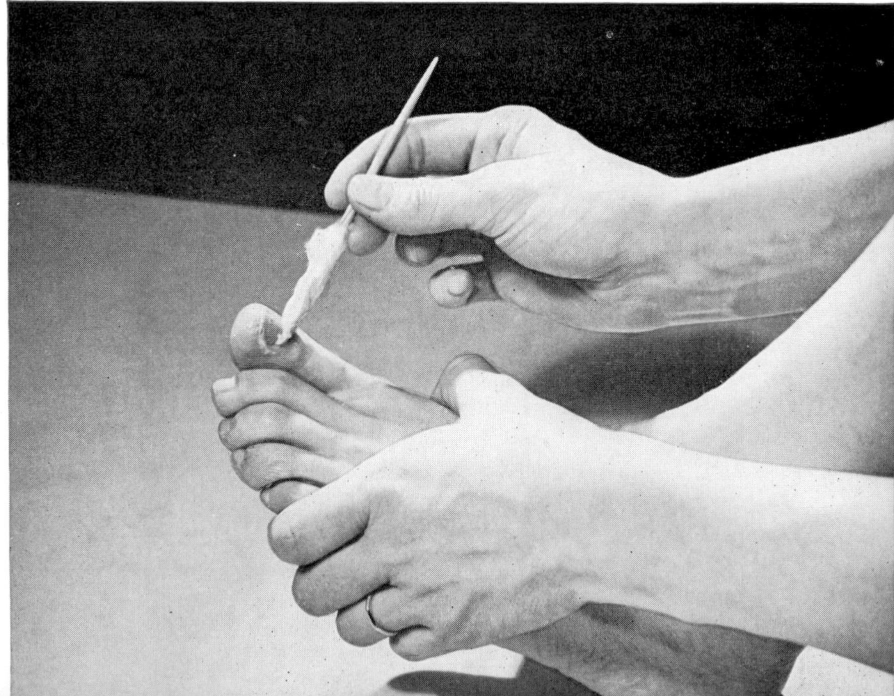

9. PERSONAL AND SOCIAL FACTORS

An Understanding of diabetes and its treatment is not complete without an awareness of the personal and social factors which are an integral part of successful treatment. Environmental circumstances create tensions and anxieties common to all whether they are related to family, friends or work associations. The more important factors include family traditions, recreation, the cost of medical care, marriage and pregnancy, and personal adjustments to environment.

NATIONALITY

Many persons will adhere to certain traditions of their own, originating primarily from their racial stock. These affect not only the choice and the preparation of food but also determine social practices and conventions. There is no need for these to be sacrificed when diabetes is present, provided that there is a thorough understanding of the flexibility of the diet and the factors other than food that determine the success of treatment so that the necessary adaptations can be accomplished.

RECREATION

The value of relaxation associated with recreation has long been recognized for everyone. Recreation can and should be accomplished with determination. Actually, every attempt should be made to participate in the social activities as was the practice prior to the onset of the diabetes. By so doing, there will be greater assurance of the continuation of a normal and enjoyable routine of living. However, one should remember that excessive fatigue can be upsetting and is to be avoided.

COST OF MEDICAL CARE

Medical care will subject the patient to extra expense, which will vary according to the type of treatment required and the frequency of visits to the physician. These expenses could be of concern, depending upon the individual's financial circumstances. There may be need for careful budgeting of other expenditures so there is no undue worry and strain resulting from the cost of medical care, medication and necessary equipment.

MARRIAGE

The successful marriage must necessarily be based upon sound and secure relationships. In married life, as in all family affairs, the individual is dependent upon those who surround him for complete family and social welfare. Therefore, when matrimony is contemplated, the prospective mate always should be informed of the diabetic condition. In addition, it is most essential to provide an understanding of the disease and its treatment so that the adjustments which are indicated in the routine events of daily life can be prepared for.

Then, too, the considerations pertaining to childbearing should be discussed fully by the two parties concerned and the physician. This matter can be discussed only generally here, since each situation needs individual attention.

PREGNANCY

Today, the chances for a successful pregnancy are more promising for the diabetic patient. However, it should be realized that the possibilities of successful pregnancies with living babies are somewhat lessened when diabetes is present. During pregnancy, there are changes in glandular secretions (hormones) with accompanying variations in the status of the diabetes. These, when combined with variable amounts of physical activity, nausea or vomiting or emotional factors, often are the cause of fluctuations in blood-sugar levels. Any one of these conditions, alone or in combination, can increase susceptibility to insulin reactions (hypoglycemia), or excessive amounts of sugar in the urine with or without accompanying acidosis.

It is generally accepted that delivery for diabetic mothers is planned a short time before the normal date of expectancy and, also, that the progeny of diabetic mothers are usually delicate at the time of birth. Therefore, close teamwork is essential between the physician, the obstetrician and the patient throughout the entire period of pregnancy, as well as directly following delivery. No less attention needs to be given the newborn infant by the pediatrician.

The careful and constant medical attention essential during pregnancy necessitates frequent visits to the physician so that the changes in the status of the diabetes can be evaluated and, when indicated, changes in treatment can be made. Usually, regardless of previous therapy for the regulation of the diabetes, the patient will require insulin, in addition to the prescribed diet. The oral hypoglycemic agents, presently available are not recommended for the management of diabetes during pregnancy. The patient will need to perform regularly the urine tests for sugar (pp. 148-162) and record the results for presentation to the physician on scheduled visits. Urine tests for acetone (pp. 163, 164) will be necessary when unduly large amounts of sugar are present in the urine.

Throughout the pregnancy there will be variations in the requirements of insulin, often to a great degree. Careful adherence to the prescribed diet is extremely important. The diet will need to be supplemented with a vitamin preparation to assure fulfillment of the increased nutritional requirement.

Although the status of the diabetes changes during the course of the pregnancy, the severity of the disease usually remains unchanged following delivery. Modern scientific knowledge concerning therapeutic measures encompassing diligent diabetic control, careful prenatal and postnatal care, as well as the handling of the newborn infant, have been largely responsible for the present degree of success in this sphere of medicine. The need for the closest co-operation of patient and physician cannot be emphasized too heavily, nor too frequently. Co-operation here, as in so many other instances, can be most rewarding in its results.

HEREDITY

There is reliable scientific information, upon which most authorities agree, that a tendency toward diabetes may be inherited as a recessive characteristic according to the Mendelian Law of Heredity. According to this theory, when only one parent has diabetes, the offsprings will seldom develop diabetes, but they will be potential carriers (having a history of diabetes in the family). When 2 hereditary carriers marry, 1 out of every 4 or 25 per cent of their children may develop the disease, and 3 out of every 4 or 75 per cent of their children will be carriers. When a person with diabetes marries a hereditary carrier, one half or 50 per cent of the offsprings are expected to develop diabetes, and one half or 50 per cent will be carriers. When 2 persons who have diabetes marry, all of their children are expected to develop diabetes.

Under any of these circumstances, diabetes does not necessarily occur during childhood, or even adolescence, but may develop later in life. (See Heredity and Expected Incidence of Diabetes, How the Mendelian Law of Heredity Applies to Parents and Their Children, page 5).

HUMAN RELATIONSHIPS

There is no greater influence upon an individual than that of his family, for relationships with the members affect the many necessary adjustments to daily routines. Although self-reliance is commendable and desirable, no one lives unto himself alone, and so the patient with diabetes must think of himself as part of his family and community as he participates in everyday activities. Environmental factors are constantly providing circumstances to which all individuals need to adapt themselves continually. As long as one has the capacity to adjust successfully to his environment, whether involved with family, friends or those at work or school, the chances of good mental and physical hygiene are enhanced.

While it is true that a diabetic patient must consider his condition seriously, there is no reason to feel that the normal channels of life are denied him, for thousands of persons with diabetes are enjoying long, useful and happy lives. The fact that there is treatment for the control of diabetes is the patient's inspiration. *Knowing this, and with wholehearted and determined effort, successful treatment can be realized.* And the information set forth in this book has been simply to provide you, the patient, with the accumulated experience for the care of your diabetes and consequently your total welfare.

APPENDIX

TABLES OF IDEAL WEIGHT

Table 15. Desirable Weights for Men and Women of Ages 25 and Over*
Weight in Pounds According to Height and Frame (In Indoor Clothing)

Men					Women				
Height (with shoes on) 1-inch heels Ft.	In.	Small Frame	Medium Frame	Large Frame	Height (with shoes on) 2-inch heels Ft.	In.	Small Frame	Medium Frame	Large Frame
5	2	112-120	118-129	126-141	4	10	92- 98	96-107	104-119
5	3	115-123	121-133	129-144	4	11	94-101	98-110	106-122
5	4	118 126	124-136	132-148	5	0	96-104	101-113	109-125
5	5	121-129	127-139	135-152	5	1	99-107	104-116	112-128
5	6	124-133	130-143	138-156	5	2	102-110	107-119	115-131
5	7	128-137	134-147	142-161	5	3	105-113	110-122	118-134
5	8	132-141	138-152	147-166	5	4	108-116	113-126	121-138
5	9	136-145	142-156	151-170	5	5	111-119	116-130	125-142
5	10	140-150	146 160	155-174	5	6	114-123	120-135	129-146
5	11	144-154	150-165	159-179	5	7	118-127	124-139	133-150
6	0	148-158	154-170	164-184	5	8	122-131	128-143	137-154
6	1	152-162	158-175	168-189	5	9	126-135	132-147	141-158
6	2	156-167	162-180	173-194	5	10	130-140	136-151	145-163
6	3	160-171	167-185	178-199	5	11	134-144	140-155	149-168
6	4	164-175	172-190	182-204	6	0	138-148	144-159	153 173

For girls between 18 and 25, subtract 1 pound for each year under 25.

* Prepared by the Metropolitan Life Insurance Company, 1960. Derived primarily from data of the Build and Blood Pressure Study, 1959, Society of Actuaries.

HEIGHT AND WEIGHT TABLES FOR BOYS AND GIRLS

The height and weight tables presented on the following pages are intended to serve as a guide for determining and evaluating growth of boys and girls from 1 to 18 years of age. Since there is considerable variation in rates of growth, the figures on the tables are given for the short, medium and tall individual in each age group. *The age and the height are the basis for obtaining the ideal or desirable weight.* For example, when the height occurs in the "short" column, the "short" column should also be used for finding desirable weight. Similarly, when the height appears in the "medium" or the "tall" column the figure for desirable weight may be found in the "medium" or the "tall column" respectively. When the height falls between the figures listed in any two columns, then approximate weights may be estimated (Tables 16 and 17).

TABLE 16. HEIGHT AND WEIGHT TABLE FOR BOYS*

(1 to 18 years of age)

AGE YEARS	HEIGHT RANGE† INCHES‡			WEIGHT RANGE ACCORDING TO HEIGHT† POUNDS‡		
	Short	Medium	Tall	Short	Medium	Tall
1	29	30	31	20	22	26
2	33	35	36	25	28	32
3	36	38	40	29	32	37
4	39	41	43	32	37	42
5	41	43	46	36	42	48
6	44	46	49	41	48	57
7	46	49	52	46	54	65
8	49	51	54	51	60	73
9	51	53	56	56	66	81
10	52	55	58	61	72	90
11	54	57	60	66	78	99
12	56	59	62	72	85	110
13	58	61	65	77	93	123
14	60	64	68	87	108	137
15	62	66	70	100	120	148
16	64	68	71	111	130	157
17	65	69	72	118	136	165
18	66	69	72	120	139	169

* Adapted from Watson and Lowrey: Growth and Development of Children, ed. 2, Chicago, Year Book Pub., 1954, Weight Percentile Table; and adapted from anthropometric charts based on original data of H. C. Stuart and H. V. Meredith and prepared for use in Children's Medical Center, Boston.

† Height without shoes and weight without clothing except for light undergarments.

‡ Figures rounded to the nearest whole number.

TABLE 17. HEIGHT AND WEIGHT TABLE FOR GIRLS*

(1 to 18 years of age)

AGE YEARS	HEIGHT RANGE† INCHES‡			WEIGHT RANGE ACCORDING TO HEIGHT† POUNDS‡		
	Short	Medium	Tall	Short	Medium	Tall
1	28	29	30	18	21	25
2	32	34	36	24	27	32
3	36	38	40	28	32	38
4	39	41	43	31	36	44
5	41	43	46	36	41	49
6	44	46	48	40	47	54
7	46	48	51	45	52	61
8	48	51	53	49	58	70
9	50	52	55	53	64	79
10	52	55	58	57	70	90
11	54	57	61	63	79	101
12	56	60	63	70	88	112
13	59	62	65	80	99	125
14	60	63	66	91	109	133
15	61	64	66	98	114	138
16	62	64	67	101	117	141
17	62	64	67	103	119	143
18	62	64	67	104	120	145

* Adapted from Watson and Lowrey: Growth and Development of Children, ed. 2, Chicago, Year Book Pub., 1954, Weight Percentile Table; and adapted from anthropometric charts based on original data of H. C. Stuart and H. V. Meredith and prepared for use in Children's Medical Center, Boston.

† Height without shoes and weight without clothing except for light undergarments.

‡ Figures rounded to the nearest whole number.

RECOMMENDED AMOUNTS OF THE FOOD NUTRIENTS

Through study and research, scientists have been able to determine how much of the various food nutrients the body requires. These amounts are measured in weights of the metric system* as grams, milligrams, micrograms and kilograms. The metric system is based on decimal measurements in 10's, 100's, 1,000's, 1,000,000's, similar to those used in our monetary system.

In this country pounds and ounces are used for weights. There are 16 ounces in a pound. When less than one ounce is used, it is called by a fraction of an ounce, such as 1/4 of an ounce. The basic measure of weight in the metric system is the gram. There are about 28 grams in one ounce. One thousand grams (1,000 times a gram) equal one kilogram. One kilogram is equal to about 2.2 pounds. When the gram is divided by 1,000 (1/1000 of a gram), the result is a milligram (*milli* meaning 1/1000). Again, when the milligram is divided by 1,000 (or the gram is divided by 1,000,000) the result is a microgram (Table 18). The microgram is easy to remember because most people are familiar with the microscope, an optical instrument used to make tiny objects visible to the naked eye.

As has been stated, the normal daily needs of the body are based on the patient's ideal or desirable weight measured in kilograms. The normal diet is figured by using certain amounts of each of the food nutrients for every kilogram of ideal body weight.

The amounts of the various food nutrients recommended at the present time for calculating the normal diet for any person for one day are shown in Table 19.

* The metric system was devised many years ago during the French Revolution, when a Commission of Scientists was appointed to simplify methods of weights and measures. This system is commonly used in all countries except the United States and Great Britain, although scientists in these countries do employ it.

TABLE 18. MEASUREMENTS OF WEIGHTS OF THE METRIC SYSTEM

28 grams (about)	= 1 ounce
1 gram	= 1,000 milligrams
1 milligram	= 1,000 micrograms
1 gram	= 1,000,000 micrograms
1 kilogram	= 1,000 grams
1 kilogram	= 2.2 pounds

The kilogram can be used in weighing people

Example: 154 pounds = 70 kilograms

132 pounds = 60 kilograms

Table 19. Recommended Daily Needs of the Body*

1 ounce = 28 grams; 1 milligram = 1/1,000 gram; 1 microgram = 1/1,000 milligram; 1 kilogram (Kg.) = 1,000 grams (2.2 lbs.)

	Carbo-hydrate†	Pro-tein	Fat†	Carbo-hydrate†	Pro-tein	Fat†
	Grams per Kilogram of Ideal Body Weight			Total Grams Figured from Ideal Weight		
ADULTS: Moderate Activity						
Man (154 lbs. = 70 kg.)	4– 6	1 –1½	1½–2	280–420	70–105	105–140
Woman (128 lbs. = 58 kg.)	4– 6	1 –1½	1 –1½	232–348	58– 87	58– 87
Pregnancy (2nd and 3rd trimester)	5– 6	1½–2	1 –2	290–348	87–116	58–116
Lactation	7– 8	1¾–2	1½–2	406–464	102–116	87–116
CHILDREN:						
1– 3 years (29 lbs. = 13 kg.)	12–14	3 –3½	3 –4	156–182	39– 46	39– 52
3– 6 years (40 lbs. = 18 kg.)	10–12	2½–3	2½–3½	180–216	45– 54	45– 63
6– 9 years (53 lbs. = 24 kg.)	8–10	2 –2½	2 –3	192–240	48– 60	48– 72
GIRLS:						
9–12 years (72 lbs. = 33 kg.)	7– 9	1¾–2	2 –3	231–297	58– 66	66– 99
12–15 years (103 lbs. = 47 kg.)	5– 7	1½–2	1½–2	235–329	71– 94	71– 94
15–18 years (117 lbs. = 53 kg.)	5– 7	1 –1½	1 –1½	265–371	53– 80	53– 80
BOYS:						
9–12 years (72 lbs. = 33 kg.)	7– 9	2 –2½	2 –3	231–297	66– 83	66– 99
12–15 years (98 lbs. = 45 kg.)	6– 8	1½–2	2 –3	270–360	68– 90	90–135
15–18 years (134 lbs. = 61 kg.)	6– 8	1½–2	2 –2½	366–488	92–122	122–153

* Adapted from Recommended Dietary Allowances of the Food and Nutrition Board of the National Research Council, 1964.

† The amounts of carbohydrate and fat must be adjusted to meet the caloric needs of the individual.

CALORIES: To estimate the total calories multiply the grams of carbohydrate and the grams of protein by 4 and the grams of fat by 9. Total the results.

TABLE 19. RECOMMENDED DAILY NEEDS OF THE BODY (*Continued*)

1 ounce = 28 grams; 1 milligram = 1/1,000 gram; 1 microgram = 1/1,000 milligram; 1 kilogram (Kg.) = 1,000 grams (2.2 lbs.)

	CALCIUM	IRON	VITAMIN A	THIAMINE	RIBOFLAVIN	NIACIN	ASCORBIC ACID	VITAMIN D
	Grams	Milligrams	International Units	Micrograms	Micrograms	Milligram Equivalents	Milligrams	International Units
ADULTS: Moderate Activity								
Man (154 lbs. = 70 kg.)	0.8	10	5,000	1,000	1,600	17	70	..
Woman (128 lbs. = 58 kg.)	0.8	15	5,000	800	1,200	13	70	..
Pregnancy (2nd and 3rd trimester)	1.3	20	6,000	1,000	1,500	16	100	400
Lactation	1.3	20	8,000	1,200	1,800	20	100	400
CHILDREN:								
1– 3 years (29 lbs. = 13 kg.)	0.8	8	2,000	500	800	9	40	400
3– 6 years (40 lbs. = 18 kg.)	0.8	10	2,500	600	1,000	11	50	400
6– 9 years (53 lbs. = 24 kg.)	0.8	12	3,500	800	1,300	14	60	400
GIRLS:								
9–12 years (72 lbs. = 33 kg.)	1.1	15	4,500	900	1,300	15	80	400
12 15 years (103 lbs. = 47 kg.)	1.3	15	5,000	1,000	1,500	17	80	400
15–18 years (117 lbs. = 53 kg.)	1.3	15	5,000	900	1,300	15	70	400
BOYS:								
9–12 years (72 lbs. = 33 kg.)	1.1	15	4,500	1,000	1,400	16	70	400
12–15 years (98 lbs. = 45 kg.)	1.4	15	5,000	1,200	1,800	20	80	400
15–18 years (134 lbs. = 61 kg.)	1.4	15	5,000	1,400	2,000	22	80	400

Table 20. Food Values

This table lists the foods commonly used in the American dietary. Not all of these foods are necessarily recommended for the diabetic diet, but they are included to indicate their values and to serve as references. For practical purposes the figures for carbohydrate, protein and fat have been rounded to the nearest whole numbers. The figures for calories listed in this table have been calculated by using the figures of 4 calories per gram of carbohydrate, 4 calories per gram of protein, and 9 calories per gram of fat rather than the more nearly accurate method used in arriving at total caloric value as described in the U. S. Department of Agriculture Handbook No. 8.

Key to Symbols: * signifies 0.5 gram or less; — signifies no value.

Sources of figures used:

Bowes, A. deP., and Church, C. E.: *Food Values of Portions Commonly Used*, ed. 10, Philadelphia, J. B. Lippincott Co., 1966.

Nutritional Values of Nabisco Products, New York, National Biscuit Co.

Rosenthal, H., Baker, P. C., and McVey, W. A.: *Stern's Applied Dietetics,* ed. 3, Baltimore, Williams and Wilkins, 1949.

Watt, B. K., and Merrill, A. L.: *Composition of Foods — Raw, Processed, Prepared* (United States Department of Agriculture Handbook No. 8) Washington, D. C., Government Printing Office, 1963.

Food	Gram Weight	Household Measure	Grams: Carbohydrate	Grams: Protein	Grams: Fat	Calories
Beverages						
Cocoa, dry powder	2	1 teaspoon	1	*	1	13
Coffee, clear	—	1 cup	1	*	*	4
Postum, Instant, clear	185	1 cup (2 rounded tablespoons Postum)	9	1	*	40
Special dietary drinks	170	1 bottle (6 ounces)	—	—	—	—
Tea, clear	—	1 cup	*	*	—	*
Water, carbonated	170	1 bottle (6 ounces)	—	—	—	—
Breads						
Bagel	65	1 whole	33	5	2	170
Biscuit, baking powder	38	1 (2½" diameter)	17	3	7	143
Boston brown bread	35	1 slice (½" thick)	16	2	*	72
Bread, cracked wheat	23	1 slice	12	2	*	56
French or Vienna	20	1 slice (1" thick)	11	2	1	61
Italian	28	1 slice (½" thick)	16	3	*	76
raisin	23	1 slice	12	2	1	65
rye, American	23	1 slice	12	2	*	56
rye, pumpernickel	32	1 slice (4½" x 3½" x ⅛")	17	3	*	80
white	23	1 slice	12	2	1	65
whole wheat	23	1 slice	11	2	1	61

FOOD	GRAM WEIGHT	HOUSEHOLD MEASURE	GRAMS Carbo-hydrate	Protein	Fat	CALORIES
Breads (*Continued*)						
Bread crumbs, dry, grated	17	3 tablespoons	13	2	1	69
Bread sticks, thin	16	4 (9" long)	12	2	*	65
Bulkie roll	39	1 whole (4" diameter)	33	5	2	170
Corn bread	24	1½" cube	11	2	1	61
Doughnut, cake type	32	1 average	16	2	6	126
English muffin	52	1 (3¼" diameter)	31	5	5	189
Muffin, plain	48	1 (2¾" diameter)	20	4	5	141
Pancake	27	1 cake (4" diameter)	9	2	2	62
Roll, frankfurter	44	1 average	22	4	1	113
hamburger	41	1 average	21	4	1	109
hard	52	1 roll	31	5	2	162
Parker House	28	1 roll	15	2	2	86
plain, pan	38	1 average	20	3	2	110
whole wheat	35	1 average	18	4	1	97
Toast, melba	15	4 slices	11	2	1	61
Waffle	75	1 (4½" x 5½" x ½")	28	7	7	203
Cereals						
Barley, dry	21	1½ tablespoons	17	2	*	76
Cheerios	19	¾ cup	13	3	1	73
Cornflakes	19	¾ cup	16	2	*	72
Corn grits, cooked	121	½ cup	13	2	*	60
Cornmeal, dry	18	2 tablespoons (½ cup cooked)	14	1	*	60
Corn, popped, plain	21	1½ cups	16	3	1	85
Cracked wheat, cooked	—	½ cup	15	2	*	68
Cream of wheat, cooked	120	½ cup	14	2	*	64
Farina, cooked	119	½ cup	10	2	*	48
Grape nuts	14	2 tablespoons	12	1	*	52
Grape-nut flakes	18	½ cup	15	2	*	68
Hominy, cooked	121	½ cup	13	2	*	60
Kix	19	¾ cup	15	2	1	77
Krumbles	18	½ cup	16	2	*	72
Maltex, cooked	120	½ cup	16	2	*	72
Muffets	23	1 biscuit	18	2	*	80
Oatmeal, cooked	118	½ cup	11	2	1	61
Puffed rice	18	1¼ cups	16	1	*	68
Puffed wheat	18	1½ cups	14	3	*	68
Ralston, cooked	—	½ cup	15	3	*	72
Rice flakes	15	½ cup	13	1	—	56
Rice Krispies	21	¾ cup	19	1	*	80
Rice, white, cooked	63	½ cup, scant	15	1	*	64
precooked, dry	16	2 tablespoons	13	1	*	56
Shredded wheat	23	1 average biscuit	18	2	*	80
Tapioca, dry	20	2 tablespoons	17	*	*	68

Table 20. Food Values *(Continued)*

Food	Gram Weight	Household Measure	Grams			Calories
			Carbo-hydrate	Protein	Fat	
Cereals (*Continued*)						
Wheat Chex	19	⅓ cup (31 biscuits)	15	2	*	68
Wheatena, cooked	—	½ cup	16	2	*	72
Wheaties	21	¾ cup	17	2	*	76
Crackers						
Animal	16	8 crackers	13	1	2	74
Arrowroot	14	3 crackers	11	1	2	66
Butter thins	16	4 crackers	11	1	2	66
Cheese Tid-Bits	14	15 pieces	9	1	2	58
Chippers, potato crackers	12	4 crackers	7	1	3	59
Cracker meal	15	1½ tablespoons	11	1	2	66
Crax	16	4 crackers	8	4	*	48
Graham	21	3 crackers	15	2	2	86
Matzoth	20	1 (6″ diameter)	17	2	*	76
Matzoth meal	18	3 tablespoons	16	*	*	64
Milk (Royal Lunch)	12	1 cracker	8	1	2	54
Oyster	16	20 crackers	11	1	2	66
Pilot (Crown)	17	1 cracker	13	1	2	74
Pretzels, thin sticks	5	5 sticks	4	*	*	16
Ritz, plain	13	4 crackers	8	1	4	72
Ritz, cheese	14	4 crackers	8	1	4	72
Ry-Krisp	19	3 double squares	14	2	*	64
Saltines	16	4 crackers	11	1	2	66
Sandwich,						
peanut butter cheese	16	2 (4 per pack)	8	2	4	76
Soda	18	3 crackers	13	2	2	78
Triangle thins	14	8 crackers	8	2	4	76
Triscuit	13	3 crackers	9	1	2	58
Uneeda	16	3 biscuits	12	2	2	74
Venus wafers	15	4 crackers	8	4	4	84
Wheat thins	14	8 crackers	10	1	3	71
Zwieback	15	2 pieces	11	2	1	61
Dairy Products						
Butter	5	1 teaspoon	*	*	4	36
Cheese, American, process	28	1 ounce	*	7	8	100
Blue or Roquefort	28	1 ounce	1	6	9	109
Camembert	28	1 ounce	*	5	7	83
Cheddar	28	1 ounce (1″ cube)	1	7	9	113
Cheddar cheese foods	28	1 ounce	2	6	7	95
Cheddar cheese spread	28	1 ounce	2	5	6	82
Cottage	57	2 rounded tablespoons	2	8	2	58
Cream	15	1 tablespoon	*	1	6	58
Edam	28	1 ounce	1	8	6	90
Limburger	28	1 ounce	1	6	8	100

TABLE 20. FOOD VALUES (*Continued*)

Food	Gram Weight	Household Measure	Grams: Carbohydrate	Grams: Protein	Grams: Fat	Calories
Dairy Products (*Continued*)						
Cheese (*Continued*)						
Parmesan, grated	28	1 ounce (4 tablespoons)	1	10	7	107
Ricotta	42	1½ ounces	*	2	5	53
Swiss	28	1 ounce	*	8	8	104
Swiss, process	28	1 ounce	*	7	8	100
Cream, all purpose	15	1 tablespoon	*	*	5	45
heavy	15	1 tablespoon	*	*	6	54
light, sweet	30	2 tablespoons	1	1	6	62
sour or cultured	30	1 ounce	1	1	5	53
whipped, unsweetened	30	2 tablespoons	*	*	6	54
Cream substitute, dried	3	1 teaspoon	2	*	1	17
Egg, whole, dried	14	2 tablespoons (equals 1 egg)	1	7	6	86
Egg, whole, fresh	50	1 large	*	7	6	82
Egg white, fresh	33	1 white	*	4	*	16
Egg yolk, fresh	17	1 yolk	*	3	5	57
Ice cream, plain	68	½ cup	13	3	7	127
Ice milk	94	½ cup	21	5	5	149
Milk, buttermilk	246	1 cup (8 ounces)	13	9	*	88
condensed, sweetened	20	1 tablespoon	11	2	2	70
dried skim, powder	21	3 tablespoons	11	8	*	76
dried whole, powder	28	4 tablespoons	11	7	8	144
evaporated, whole	126	½ cup (4 ounces)	12	9	10	174
goat's	244	1 cup (8 ounces)	11	8	10	166
skim, cow's	246	1 cup (8 ounces)	13	9	*	88
whole, cow's	30	2 tablespoons	2	1	1	21
whole, cow's	244	1 cup (8 ounces)	12	9	9	165
Malted milk powder, plain	9	1 tablespoon	6	1	1	37
Yoghurt, plain	246	1 cup	12	7	8	148
Desserts						
Cookie, plain	25	1 cookie (3″ diameter)	18	1	5	121
Cake, angel food	45	1/10 average cake	27	3	*	120
plain	55	1 piece (3″ x 2″ x 1½″)	31	3	8	208
sponge	50	1/10 average cake	27	4	3	151
Custard, baked	124	½ cup	14	7	7	147
Gelatin, plain, dry	10	1 tablespoon	—	9	—	36
Ice cream, plain	68	½ cup	13	3	7	127
Ice cream cone	12	1 cone (no ice cream)	9	1	*	40
Jello, plain, ready to eat	120	½ cup	17	2	—	76
Fats and Oils						
Bacon fat	5	1 teaspoon	—	—	5	45
Blue cheese or Roquefort dressing	16	1 tablespoon	1	1	8	80

Table 20. Food Values *(Continued)*

Food	Gram Weight	Household Measure	Grams: Carbo-hydrate	Grams: Protein	Grams: Fat	Calories
Fats and Oils *(Continued)*						
Butter	5	1 teaspoon	*	*	4	36
Chicken fat	5	1 teaspoon	—	—	5	45
Chocolate, unsweetened, melted	8	2 teaspoons	2	1	4	48
Cooking fat or shortening	4	1 teaspoon	—	—	4	36
French dressing	15	1 tablespoon	3	*	6	66
Gravy, brown	—	2 tablespoons	2	*	4	44
Italian dressing	14	1 tablespoon	1	*	8	76
Italian tomato sauce, plain	—	¼ cup	5	1	5	69
Lard	5	1 teaspoon	—	—	5	45
Margarine	5	1 teaspoon	*	*	4	36
Mayonnaise	8	1 full teaspoon	*	*	6	54
Oils, salad or cooking	5	1 teaspoon	—	—	5	45
Peanut butter	11	2 teaspoons	2	3	5	65
Salad dressing, mayonnaise type	15	1 tablespoon	2	*	6	62
Salt pork	5	¾″ cube	—	*	4	36
Tartar sauce	7	1 teaspoon	*	*	4	36
White sauce, medium	33	2 tablespoons	3	1	4	52
Fish, cooked or canned						
Anchovies	28	7 thin fillets	*	5	3	47
Clams	50	5 medium	1	1	8	80
Crab	43	¼ cup, flaked	*	8	1	41
Cod, fresh	28	1 ounce	—	8	2	50
dried, salted	28	1 ounce	—	8	*	32
Fish sticks, frozen	114	5 sticks	7	19	10	194
Flounder	28	1 ounce	—	8	2	50
Haddock	28	1 ounce	—	7	*	28
Halibut	28	1 ounce	—	7	2	46
Herring, lake	28	1 ounce	—	7	1	37
pickled	28	1 ounce	—	6	4	60
smoked, kippered	28	1 ounce	—	6	4	60
Lobster	43	¼ cup	*	8	1	41
Mackerel	28	1 ounce	—	7	5	73
Oysters	57	5 medium	3	6	1	45
Salmon	28	1 ounce (¼ cup, flaked)	—	8	2	50
Sardines	28	1 ounce (2 medium)	—	7	3	55
Scallops, bay or sea	28	1 ounce (1 piece, 12 per pound)	—	7	*	28
Shrimp	28	3 large or 5 medium	*	7	*	28
Swordfish	28	1 ounce	—	7	2	46
Trout, brook	28	1 ounce	—	7	1	37
Tuna, canned, drained	28	¼ cup, flaked	—	8	2	50
Whitefish	28	1 ounce	—	7	3	55

TABLE 20. FOOD VALUES *(Continued)*

FOOD	GRAM WEIGHT	HOUSEHOLD MEASURE	GRAMS Carbo-hydrate	Protein	Fat	CALORIES
Flour and Flour Products						
Cornstarch	16	2 tablespoons	14	*	*	56
Flour, white	16	2 tablespoons	12	2	*	56
Macaroni	49	½ cup, scant	15	2	*	68
Noodles, chow mein	18	½ cup	10	2	4	84
Noodles, egg	60	½ cup, scant	14	3	1	77
Spaghetti	49	½ cup, scant	15	2	*	68
Fruit,* unsweetened						
Apple	—	1 small (2″ diameter)	12	*	*	48
Apple	75	½ medium (2½″ diameter)	9	*	*	36
Applesauce	120	½ cup	13	*	*	52
Apricots, fresh	75	2 whole	9	*	*	36
canned, waterpack	100	3 medium halves	10	1	*	44
dried, uncooked	15	4 small halves	10	1	*	44
Avocado, raw	25	⅛ (3¼″ x 4″)	2	*	4	44
Banana	75	½ (6″ long)	11	1	*	48
Blackberries, fresh	72	½ cup	9	1	1	49
canned, waterpack	100	½ cup, scant	9	1	1	49
Blueberries, fresh	70	½ cup	11	*	*	44
canned, waterpack	121	½ cup	12	1	*	52
frozen, no sugar	80	½ cup	11	1	*	48
Cantaloupe or muskmelon	—	¼ (6″ diameter)	15	1	*	64
Cherries, sweet, raw	—	10 large or 17 small	12	1	*	52
canned, waterpack	100	½ cup, scant	12	1	*	52
Cranberries, cooked	85	½ cup	9	*	1	45
Cranberry sauce, regular strained	35	1 rounded tablespoon	13	—	*	52
Currants, red or white, raw	100	¾ cup	12	1	*	52
Dates, natural and dried	20	2 medium	15	*	*	60
Figs, raw	42	1 medium	9	*	*	36
canned, waterpack	100	3 medium	12	*	*	48
dried	20	1 medium	14	1	*	60
Fruit cocktail, waterpack	100	½ cup, scant	10	*	*	40
Grapefruit, fresh	190	½ small (3⅞″ diameter)	13	*	*	52
canned, waterpack	120	½ cup	10	1	*	44
Grapes, American varieties	—	15 medium	10	1	1	53
green seedless	67	40 grapes	11	*	*	44
Honeydew melon	—	¼ small (5″ diameter)	8	1	*	36
Lemon or lime	106	1 medium	6	1	*	28
Loganberries, fresh	75	½ cup	11	1	*	48

* Figures for all canned fruit include solids and liquid.

TABLE 20. FOOD VALUES *(Continued)*

Food	Gram Weight	Household Measure	Grams: Carbo-hydrate	Grams: Protein	Grams: Fat	Calories
Fruit *(Continued)*						
Muskmelon	—	¼ (6″ diameter)	15	1	*	64
Nectarine	—	1 medium	9	*	*	36
Olives, green or ripe	64	7 large	1	*	7	67
Orange	150	1 small (2½″ diameter)	12	1	*	52
Peach, fresh	114	1 medium (2″ diameter)	10	1	*	44
canned, waterpack	123	½ cup	10	*	*	40
Pear, fresh	—	1 small	15	1	*	64
Pear, fresh	91	½ medium	13	*	*	52
canned, waterpack	117	2 medium halves	10	*	*	40
Persimmon, Japanese, raw	63	½ (2½″ diameter)	10	*	*	40
Pineapple, fresh	84	1 slice (3½″ x ¾″)	12	*	*	48
fresh, diced	70	½ cup	10	*	*	40
canned, waterpack	100	1 large slice	10	*	*	40
Plums, fresh	120	2 medium	14	*	*	56
Pomegranate, raw, pulp and seeds	50	½ medium	8	*	*	32
Prunes, dried, uncooked	16	2 medium	9	*	*	36
cooked	30	2 plus 2 teaspoons liquid	9	*	*	36
Raisins, dried, seedless	15	1 full tablespoon	12	*	*	48
Raspberries, fresh, black	67	½ cup	11	1	1	57
red	62	½ cup	8	1	*	36
Rhubarb, cubed	244	2 cups raw or 1 cup cooked	9	2	*	44
Strawberries, fresh	130	13 large	11	1	1	57
Tangerine	114	1 medium (2½″ diameter)	10	1	*	44
Watermelon	345	½ slice (10″ x ¾″)	11	1	*	48
cubes or balls	150	¾ cup	11	1	*	48
Fruit Juices, unsweetened						
Apple	83	⅓ cup	10	*	*	40
Apricot	47	⅓ cup	12	*	*	48
Grapefruit, canned and frozen (diluted 1:3)	124	½ cup	12	1	*	52
Grape, bottled or canned	64	¼ cup	11	*	*	44
Lemon, fresh	185	¾ cup	15	1	*	64
bottled or canned	184	¾ cup	14	1	*	60
Lime, fresh	185	¾ cup	17	1	*	72
Orange, fresh	124	½ cup	13	1	*	56
canned	125	½ cup	14	1	*	60
frozen (diluted 1:3)	124	½ cup	13	1	*	56
Orange-grapefruit blend, canned or frozen (diluted 1:3)	125	½ cup	13	1	*	56
Pineapple, canned	83	⅓ cup	11	*	*	44

TABLE 20. FOOD VALUES *(Continued)*

FOOD	GRAM WEIGHT	HOUSEHOLD MEASURE	GRAMS Carbo-hydrate	Protein	Fat	CALORIES
Fruit Juices *(Continued)*						
Prune, bottled or canned	64	¼ cup	12	*	*	48
Tangerine, canned	124	½ cup	13	1	*	56
Tomato, bottled or canned	121	½ cup	5	1	*	24
Meat, cooked†						
Bacon, cooked,drained	8	1 full strip	*	2	4	44
Bacon, Canadian, cooked, drained	21	1 slice	*	6	4	60
Beef, chuck, pot roasted	112	4 ounces	—	29	27	359
hamburger, lean	112	4 ounces	—	31	13	241
roast, rib	112	4 ounces	—	22	44	484
roast, rump	112	4 ounces	—	26	31	383
steak, round	112	4 ounces	—	32	17	281
steak, club	112	4 ounces	—	23	46	506
Beef, canned						
corned beef	28	1 slice (3″ x 2″ x ¼″)	—	7	2	46
corned beef hash	173	¾ cup	19	15	20	316
Beef, dried or chipped, uncooked	28	2 thin slices (4″ x 5″)	—	10	2	58
Bologna	28	1 slice (4$\frac{1}{10}$″ x $\frac{1}{10}$″)	*	3	8	84
Cervelat, soft	30	1 slice (3¾″ x $\frac{3}{16}$″)	*	6	7	87
Frankfurter	51	1 (7-9 per pound)	1	6	14	154
Ham, cured	112	4 ounces	—	23	25	317
sliced	28	1 ounce	—	5	5	65
Ham, fresh	112	4 ounces	—	27	30	378
Ham, deviled, canned	20	1 rounded tablespoon	—	3	7	75
Heart, beef	112	4 ounces	1	35	6	198
Kidney, beef	112	4 ounces	1	37	13	269
Lamb, chop with bone	137	1 thick chop	—	25	33	397
leg	112	4 ounces (4 slices, 3″ x 2¾″ x ⅛″)	—	28	21	301
shoulder	112	4 ounces (4 slices, 3″ x 2¾″ x ⅛″)	—	24	31	375
Liver, beef	57	2 ounces	4	15	3	103
calf	57	2 ounces	3	15	4	108
chicken	60	2 medium	2	16	3	99
lamb	57	2 ounces	2	16	3	99
pork	57	2 ounces	2	16	3	99
Liverwurst	30	1 slice (3″x ¼″)	1	4	8	92
Minced ham	28	1 ounce	1	4	5	65
Pork, chop, with bone	98	1 thick chop	—	16	21	253
loin	112	4 ounces	—	29	28	368
Salami, cooked	30	1 slice (3¾″ x ¼″)	*	5	8	92

† Unless otherwise specified these meats have been baked, boiled, broiled or roasted without added fat or oil.

Table 20. Food Values (*Continued*)

Food	Gram Weight	Household Measure	Grams: Carbo-hydrate	Grams: Protein	Grams: Fat	Calories
Meat (*Continued*)						
dry	30	1 slice (3¾" x ¼")	*	7	11	127
Sausage, pork, links	20	1 link (3" x ½")	*	4	9	97
Polish style	30	1 slice (1" x 1½" diameter)	*	5	8	92
Tongue, canned	20	1 slice (3" x 2" x ⅛")	*	4	4	52
Veal, loin, chop	112	4 ounces	—	30	15	255
chuck	112	4 ounces	—	31	14	250
cutlet	112	4 ounces	—	30	12	228
roast, rib	112	4 ounces	—	31	19	295
Miscellaneous						
Beef and vegetable stew	235	1 cup	15	15	10	210
Catsup or chili sauce	17	1 tablespoon	4	*	*	16
Chocolate, bitter or baking	28	1 square	8	3	15	179
Chop suey (meat), canned	225	1 cup	10	10	7	143
Chow mein (chicken), canned	222	1 cup	16	6	*	88
Chili con carne, canned with beans	230	1 cup	28	17	14	306
Cocoa, dry, average	2	1 teaspoon	1	*	1	13
Cole slaw	63	½ cup	5	1	5	69
Gelatin, plain, dry	10	1 tablespoon	—	9	—	36
Gravy, brown	30	2 tablespoons	2	*	4	44
Hash, corned beef, canned	173	¾ cup	19	15	20	316
Horseradish, prepared	15	1 tablespoon	1	*	—	4
Macaroni and cheese, baked	220	1 cup	44	19	24	468
Mustard, prepared, brown	5	1 teaspoon	*	*	*	*
Pancake	54	2 (4" diameter)	18	4	4	124
Pickle, dill or sour	135	1 large (4" x 1¾")	3	1	*	16
Pizza with cheese topping	75	5½" sector or ⅛ of 14" diameter pie	21	9	6	174
Potato chips	30	15 medium (2" diameter)	15	2	12	176
Potatoes, French fried	29	5 pieces (2" x ½" x ½")	10	1	4	80
Sherbet, average	96	½ cup	29	1	—	120
Stuffing, bread, moist	63	⅓ cup	12	3	8	132
Vinegar	15	1 tablespoon	1	—	—	4
Waffle	75	1 (4½" x 5½" x ½")	28	7	7	203
White sauce, medium	66	¼ cup	6	3	8	108
Yeast cake	12	1 cake	1	2	*	12
Yeast, dried	8	1 tablespoon	3	3	*	24
Nuts						
Almonds	15	12-15 nuts	3	3	8	96
Brazil nuts	15	4 medium nuts	2	2	10	106

TABLE 20. FOOD VALUES *(Continued)*

FOOD	GRAM WEIGHT	HOUSEHOLD MEASURE	GRAMS Carbo-hydrate	Protein	Fat	CALORIES
Nuts *(Continued)*						
Cashew nuts	15	6-8 nuts	4	3	7	91
Coconut, fresh meat	15	1 piece (1″ x 1″ x ⅜″)	1	*	5	49
shredded, dried, sweetened	15	2 tablespoons	8	*	6	86
Filberts or hazelnuts		10-12 nuts	3	2	9	101
Peanuts, roasted and salted	15	15 nuts	3	4	8	100
Peanut butter	65	¼ cup	11	18	32	404
Pecans	15	12 halves or 2 tablespoons chopped	2	1	11	111
Pistachio nuts	15	30 nuts	3	3	8	96
Walnuts, English	15	8-15	2	2	10	106
Poultry, cooked						
Chicken breast, with bone, fried	94	½ breast (3³⁄₁₀ ounces)	1	25	5	149
Chicken, drumstick, with bone, fried	59	1 (2¹⁄₁₀ ounces)	*	12	4	84
Chicken, roasted, dark meat	112	4 ounces	—	33	7	195
light meat	112	4 ounces	—	36	6	198
Chicken, canned, boneless	28	1 ounce (2 tablespoons)	—	6	3	51
Duck	105	3 slices (3½″ x 2½″ x ¼″)	—	24	25	321
Goose	112	4 ounces	—	38	11	251
Turkey, dark meat	112	4 ounces	—	34	9	217
light meat	112	4 ounces	—	37	4	184
Soups, Condensed, Canned (before liquid has been added)						
Beef	156	½ can	12	14	4	140
Beef broth, bouillon or consommé	149	½ can	3	6	—	36
Beef noodle	149	½ can	9	5	3	83
Black bean	163	½ can	20	8	2	130
Chicken gumbo	149	½ can	9	4	2	70
Chicken noodle	149	½ can	10	4	2	74
Chicken rice	151	½ can	7	4	2	62
Chicken vegetable	152	½ can	12	5	3	95
Clam chowder, Manhattan style	154	½ can	15	3	3	99
Cream of asparagus	149	½ can	13	3	2	82
Cream of celery	149	½ can	11	2	6	106
Cream of chicken	149	½ can	10	4	7	119
Cream of mushroom	149	½ can	13	3	12	172
Green split pea	153	½ can	26	11	4	184
Minestrone	149	½ can	17	6	4	128
Onion	149	½ can	6	7	3	79

Table 20. Food Values *(Continued)*

Food	Gram Weight	Household Measure	Grams: Carbo-hydrate	Grams: Protein	Grams: Fat	Calories
Soups *(Continued)*						
Scotch broth	153	½ can	13	7	4	116
Tomato	153	½ can	19	2	3	111
Turkey noodle	149	½ can	10	5	4	96
Vegetable beef	156	½ can	12	7	3	103
Vegetarian vegetable	153	½ can	16	3	3	103
Soups, Condensed, Frozen (before liquid has been added)						
Clam chowder, New England style	146	½ can	13	5	9	153
Cream of potato	146	½ can	15	4	6	130
Cream of shrimp	142	½ can	10	6	14	190
Green pea with ham	149	½ can	24	11	3	167
Oyster stew	142	½ can	10	7	9	149
Soups, Dehydrated (reconstituted—after liquid has been added according to directions on package)						
Beef noodle	251	1 cup	12	3	1	69
Chicken noodle	246	1 cup	8	2	2	58
Chicken rice	246	1 cup	9	1	1	49
Green pea	251	1 cup	21	8	2	134
Onion	243	1 cup	6	2	1	41
Tomato vegetable with noodles	250	1 cup	13	2	2	78
Vegetables‡						
Artichokes, French or globe, cooked	100	1 (base and soft ends)	10	3	*	52
Asparagus, fresh, cooked	100	⅔ cup (cut pieces)	4	2	*	24
canned	96	6 spears	3	2	*	20
frozen, cooked	100	6 spears	4	3	*	28
Bamboo shoots, raw	100	¾ cup	5	3	*	32
Beans, kidney, cooked	63	¼ cup	14	5	*	76
lima, cooked	64	½ cup, scant	13	5	*	72
Navy or pea, canned with pork and molasses	47	2 full tablespoons	10	3	2	70
snap, green, cooked	125	1 cup	7	2	*	36
snap, yellow or wax, cooked	125	1 cup	6	2	*	32
Bean sprouts, mung, cooked	100	1 cup	5	3	*	32
Beets, red, cooked	124	¾ cup, diced	9	1	*	40
Beet greens, cooked	73	½ cup	2	1	*	12
Broccoli, cooked	150	1 cup	7	5	*	48
Brussels sprouts, cooked	130	1 cup (9 medium)	8	6	*	56

‡ Values for canned and frozen cooked vegetables are similar to those of cooked vegetables.

Table 20. Food Values *(Continued)*

Food	Gram Weight	Household Measure	Grams: Carbohydrate	Grams: Protein	Grams: Fat	Calories
Vegetables *(Continued)*						
Cabbage, raw	50	½ cup, shredded	3	1	*	12
cooked	170	1 cup	7	2	*	36
Carrot, raw	100	1 large	10	1	*	44
cooked	145	1 cup, diced	10	1	*	44
Cauliflower, cooked	120	1 cup	5	3	*	32
Celery, raw	40	1 stalk (8″ x 1½″ at root end)	2	*	*	8
Chard, Swiss, cooked	88	½ cup	3	2	*	20
Chicory (also called French or Belgian endive)	25	10 small inner leaves	1	*	*	4
Chick peas or garbanzos, dried, uncooked	25	2 tablespoons	15	5	1	89
Collards, cooked	143	¾ cup	7	5	1	57
Corn, fresh, cooked	140	1 small ear (5″ x 1¾″)	16	3	1	85
canned, whole kernel	83	½ cup	16	2	1	81
Cowpeas, cooked	60	½ cup, scant	11	5	*	64
Cucumber, pared, raw	50	6 slices (2″ x ⅛″)	2	*	*	8
Dandelion greens, cooked	135	¾ cup	9	3	1	57
Eggplant, cooked	100	½ cup	4	1	*	20
Endive, curly, raw	57	2 ounces	2	1	*	12
Kale, cooked	55	½ cup	3	3	*	24
Lentils, dried, cooked	56	½ cup, scant	11	4	*	60
Lettuce	50	4 small leaves	2	*	*	8
Mushrooms, raw	50	5 small	2	1	*	12
canned	122	½ cup	3	2	*	20
Mustard greens, cooked	70	½ cup	3	2	*	20
Okra, cooked	85	8 pods (3″ x ⅝″)	5	2	*	28
Onions, raw	10	1 tablespoon, chopped	1	*	*	4
cooked	210	¾ cup	10	2	*	48
Parsley, fresh	4	1 tablespoon, chopped	*	*	*	*
Parsnip, cooked	78	½ cup	12	1	*	52
Peas, dried, split, cooked	—	½ cup, scant	14	6	*	80
Peas, green, cooked	80	½ cup	10	4	*	56
canned	60	½ cup, scant	10	3	*	52
frozen, cooked	80	½ cup	9	4	*	52
Pepper, green, raw	62	1 medium pod	3	1	*	16
cooked	65	1 medium pod	3	1	*	16
Pepper, red, raw	60	1 medium pod	4	1	*	20
Pimento, canned	38	1 medium pod	2	*	*	8
Potato, sweet, baked	55	½ medium	18	1	*	76
white, boiled	100	1 small	15	2	*	68
Pumpkin, cooked	125	½ cup	10	1	*	44
Radishes, raw	40	4 small	1	*	*	4
Rutabagas, cooked	116	¾ cup, cubed	10	1	*	44

TABLE 20. FOOD VALUES *(Continued)*

FOOD	GRAM WEIGHT	HOUSEHOLD MEASURE	GRAMS Carbo-hydrate	Protein	Fat	CALORIES
Vegetables (*Continued*)						
Sauerkraut, canned, solids and liquid	118	½ cup	5	1	*	24
Spinach, cooked	90	½ cup	3	3	*	24
Squash, summer, cooked	105	½ cup, diced	3	1	*	16
winter, cooked	114	½ cup	11	1	*	48
Tomato, raw	150	1 medium (2″ x 2½″)	7	2	*	36
canned	121	½ cup	5	1	*	24
juice, bottled or canned	121	½ cup	5	1	*	24
paste, canned	32	2 tablespoons	6	1	*	28
Turnips, cooked	155	1 cup, diced	8	1	*	36
Turnip greens, cooked	73	½ cup	3	2	*	20
Vegetable juice cocktail	125	½ cup	5	1	*	24
Vegetables, mixed, frozen, cooked	75	½ cup	10	2	*	48
Water chestnuts, Chinese	25	4 chestnuts	5	*	*	20
Watercress, raw	10	10 sprigs	*	*	*	*
Zucchini, cooked	105	½ cup, diced	3	1	*	16

Table 21. Amounts of Carbohydrate, Alcohol and Calories in Alcoholic Beverages*

Alcoholic Beverage	Amount: Cubic Centimeters (cc.)	Amount: Household Measure	Grams: Alcohol†	Grams: Carbohydrate‡	Total Calories
Ale, mild	240	1 glass (8 ounces)	9	8	95
Beer, average	240	1 glass (8 ounces)	9	11	107
Brandy or Cognac	30	1 pony (1 ounce)	11	—	77
Cider, fermented	180	1 glass (6 ounces)	9	2	71
Cordials					
Anisette	20	1 cordial glass (⅔ ounce)	7	7	77
Apricot Brandy	20	1 cordial glass (⅔ ounce)	6	6	66
Benedictine	20	1 cordial glass (⅔ ounce)	7	7	77
Creme de Menthe	20	1 cordial glass (⅔ ounce)	7	6	73
Gin, dry	45	1 jigger (1½ ounces)	15	—	105
Rum	45	1 jigger (1½ ounces)	15	—	105
Whiskey					
Rye	45	1 jigger (1½ ounces)	17	—	119
Scotch	45	1 jigger (1½ ounces)	15	—	105
Wine					
Champagne	120	1 glass (4 ounces)	11	3	89
Muscatel or Port	105	1 wine glass (3½ ounces)	15	14	161
Sauterne, California	105	1 wine glass (3½ ounces)	11	4	93
Sherry	60	1 sherry glass (2 ounces)	9	5	83
Vermouth, dry	105	1 wine glass (3½ ounces)	15	1	109
Vermouth, sweet	105	1 wine glass (3½ ounces)	18	12	174

* Figures obtained from Bowes, A. deP., and Church, C. E.: *Food Values of Portions Commonly Used*, ed. 10, Philadelphia, J. B. Lippincott Co., 1966.

† Grams of alcohol are multiplied by 7 to obtain total calories.

‡ Grams of carbohydrate are multiplied by 4 to obtain total calories.

DIET CALCULATION SHEET

This page has been provided for the calculation of the diet. Space is allowed for adding the amounts of carbohydrate, protein and fat supplied by the foods eaten in one day. The food values for carbohydrate, protein and fat are found in the exchange lists. When the total amounts of these have been figured, they can then be compared with the diet prescription.

Table 22. Diet Calculation Sheet

Food	Amount	Grams		
		Carbohydrate	Protein	Fat
Milk, whole				
Milk, skimmed				
Milk, evaporated				
Cheese, American				
Cheese, cottage				
Egg				
Meat				
Fish				
Poultry				
Butter				
Other fats or oils				
Fruit: (1)				
(2)				
(3)				
(4)				
Vegetables: Group A (1)				
(2)				
Group B (1)				
(2)				
Bread or Exchange: (1)				
(2)				
(3)				
(4)				
(5)				
(6)				
Other Foods: (1)				
(2)				
(3)				
(4)				
	Totals:			
		×4	×4	×9
	Calories:			
	Total Calories:			

GLOSSARY

acetohexamide (ă-se'-tō-hĕk'-să-mīd). See Dymelor.
acetone (ăs'-et-ōn). A colorless liquid with peculiar odor and burning taste. Acetone is formed in the process of normal fat metabolism. It often appears in the urine when fat is burned improperly, as in uncontrolled diabetes.
acidosis (ăs-ĭ-dō'-sĭs), **diabetic.** Acid intoxication which results when sugar cannot be utilized in the body and fat is called upon to supply the body's need for energy, with a resultant accumulation of diacetic acid and acetone (ketone bodies).
ascorbic acid (â-skôr'-bik, ăs'-id). Vitamin C, which is needed in the body for normal development and nutrition of bones, teeth, and gums. It also helps to build and maintain the strength of the walls of the small blood vessels. Ascorbic acid is found principally in fruits and raw vegetables.

biguanides (bī-gwă'-nīdz). See DBI and DBI-ID.

calcium (kăl'-sĭ-ŭm). A food constituent needed by the body for the formation of strong bones and teeth, and essential to the needs of the heart, the nerves and the muscles. Calcium is found principally in dairy products.
calorie (kăl'-ô-rĭ). A unit for the measurement of heat; used to express the heat-producing or energy-producing value of food.
carbohydrate (kär'bō-hī'-drāt). A food constituent: the sugar and starches which provide the body with energy. Each gram of carbohydrate supplies four calories.
carrier (kă'-rĭ-ĕr). Of diabetes, a person who has a history of diabetes in his family.
chlorpropamide (klôr-prō'-pă-mīd). See Diabenese.
coma (ko'mah), **diabetic.** Loss of consciousness which results when acidosis becomes very severe.
concentrated sweets. Foods such as sugar, honey, marmalade, jam, conserve, frosting, candy and soft drinks.
controlled diabetes. The condition of diabetes where weight is maintained at an ideal level, absence of symptoms, blood-sugar levels within limits of safety, little to no sugar in the urine, and absence of acidosis or reactions.

DBI (phenformin). The brand name of an oral drug which is used in the treatment of diabetes.
DBI-TD (phenformin-timed disintegration). Brand name of an oral drug used in the treatment of diabetes.
diabetes (dī'-a-bē'-têz). A condition in which the body is unable to use and store carbohydrate normally due to an insufficient supply of insulin or to interference with the action of insulin in the body.
Diabinese (dī-ă'bĭn-ēse). (chlorpropamide) Brand name of an oral drug used in the treatment of diabetes.
dietetic foods. Foods which have been prepared commercially for special diets, such as foods packed in water without sugar, foods prepared with artificial sweetening, foods prepared without added salt, foods with mineral oil in place of fat, and others.

digestion (dĭ-jĕs′-chŭn). Process of breaking down and dissolving food chemically through the action of various secretions in the body.

Dymelor (dī′-mĕl-ôr). (acetohexamide) Brand name of an oral drug used in the treatment of diabetes.

exchanges, food. The substitution or trading of one food for another having the same food value.

fasting blood sugar. The amount of sugar contained in the blood taken before breakfast when no food has been eaten after midnight.

fat. A food constituent which is found in "fatty" foods and provides the body with energy. Each gram of fat supplies nine calories.

globin (glō′-bĭn) **insulin.** A clear amber solution of insulin which contains globin (a protein derived from hemoglobin) in addition to insulin.

Glucose Tolerance Test (glōō′-kōs, tŏl′-ĕr-ăns). A test to determine an individual's ability to use and store sugar. It consists in giving the patient a certain amount of sugar and examining the blood and urine for sugar at definite intervals.

glycogen (glī′-kô-jĕn). A form of carbohydrate which is stored in the liver and reconverted into glucose as the body has need of it.

gram (grăm). A weight of the metric system representing 1/30th of an ounce (30 grams = 1 ounce).

hereditary (hê-rĕd′-i-tĕr-ĭ). Capable of being passed by (or through) parents to offspring (e.g. diabetes).

hypoglycemia (hī-pō-glī-sē′-mē-ah). A condition in which the amount of sugar in the blood is lower than normal.

ideal weight. The desired weight of an individual which is determined according to sex, height, and body build.

insulin (in′-sū-lin). The active principle of the internal secretion of the Islets of Langerhans in the pancreas. Insulin is necessary to enable the body to use and store sugar.

iron. A food constituent which is responsible for the color and condition of the blood. It is found principally in eggs, liver, lean meat, leafy and green vegetables.

Islands of Langerhans (lahn′g-er-hans). Small groups or clusters of cells within the tissue of the pancreas, named for the German scientist, Langerhans, who first called attention to these cells.

kilogram (kĭl′-ô-grăm). A measure in the metric system which equals 2.2 pounds.

lente insulin (lĕn′-tē). A cloudy, milky-appearing insulin containing insulin and zinc.

meal plan. The suggested arrangement of the diet into meals, usually with a specified time.

Mendel's law (mĕn′-dĕlz). A law of inherited characteristics, discovered by Gregor J. Mendel, an Austrian naturalist.

metric system (mĕt′-rĭk). A decimal system of measures and weights with the meter and gram as bases. One meter = 3.28 feet. One kilogram = 2.2 pounds.

microgram (mī′-krô-grăm). A measure in the metric system, representing 1/1000 of a milligram (1,000 micrograms = 1 milligram).

milligram (mĭl′ĭ-grăm). A measure in the metric system, representing 1/1000 of a gram (1,000 milligrams = 1 gram).

niacin (nī′-ȧ-sĭn). A food constituent (member of the vitamin B complex) which helps to keep nerves and body tissue healthy. It is found principally in meat, poultry, whole grain and enriched breads and cereals, and peanuts.

obesity (ô-bēs′-ĭ-tĭ). An excessive accumulation of fat in the body.

oral hypoglycemic agents (hī-pō-glī-cē′-mĭc). Drugs which when taken by mouth lower blood-sugar levels.

Orinase (ŏr′-ĭn-ās). (tolbutamide) Brand name of an oral drug used in the treatment of diabetes.

pancreas (păn′-krē-ăs). A gland in the upper abdomen which secretes into the intestine digestive juices which act upon carbohydrate, protein and fat. It also contains the islands of Langerhans which secrete the hormone insulin.

phenformin (fĕn-fôr′mĭn). See DBI.

phenformin–timed disintegration. See DBI-TD.

polydipsia (pol-e-dip′-se-ah). Excessive thirst.

polyphagia (pol-e-fa′-je-ah). Excessive hunger.

polyuria (pol-e-ū′-re-ah). The passing of an excessive quantity of urine.

protamine-zinc insulin (pro-tam′-in). A cloudy insulin which contains insulin plus zinc and a simple protein to lengthen the action of insulin in the body.

protective diet. A diet which contains proper amounts of carbohydrate, protein, fat, minerals and vitamins.

protein (pro′-te-in). A food constituent essential to growth, building of muscle and repair of tissue. It is found principally in animal foods such as dairy products, meat and fish, and vegetables such as peas and beans, and nuts.

protein, complete. Protein containing the essential amino acids, found usually in animal sources such as milk, cheese, eggs and meat.

protein, incomplete. Protein which does not contain all of the essential amino acids, and is found usually in vegetables, grains and nuts.

reaction, insulin (rē-ăk′-shŭn). A condition which results when the blood-sugar level falls to lower than normal levels due to too much insulin or too little food.

recommended daily needs. The amounts of the various food constituents suggested by the National Research Council as being necessary for the maintenance of good health.

riboflavin (rī′bō-flā′-vĭn). A food constituent (member of the vitamin B complex) which is necessary for growth, eyesight, and healthy skin and takes part in the burning of carbohydrate. It is found principally in dairy products, meat, and green, leafy vegetables.

saccharine (săk′-ah-rĭn). A coal-tar crystalline product, several times sweeter than sugar but having no food value.

sodium chloride. Table salt.

Sulfonylurea (sŭl-fŏ-nĭl-you-rē′ă) compounds. See Orinase, Diabinese, Dymelor, Tolinase.

thiamine (thī′ȧ-mĭn). A food constituent (member of the vitamin B complex) necessary to maintain and stimulate the appetite, aid bowel movement, keep nerves and muscles healthy; it helps in the burning of carbohydrate. It is found principally in whole grain and enriched breads and cereals, meat, and vegetables.

tolazamide (tōl-ă′-ză-mīd). See Tolinase.

tolbutamide (tōl-byōō′-tă-mīd). See Orinase.

Tolinase (tōl′ĭn-ās). (tolazamide) Brand name of an oral drug used in the treatment of diabetes.

twenty-four-hour urine specimen. Sample from the total amount of urine passed in a 24-hour period.

unrestricted foods. Foods which contain no appreciable amounts of carbohydrate, protein, and fat and may be used freely in a diabetic diet unless restricted by the presence of conditions other than diabetes.

urinalysis (ū′-rĭ-năl′-ĭ-sĭs). Chemical analysis of the urine.

PERSONAL INFORMATION

PATIENT:

Name____

Address______________________________________

Telephone Number________________________________

PHYSICIAN, HOSPITAL OR CLINIC:

Name____

Address______________________________________

Telephone Number________________________________

DIET PRESCRIPTION:

Carbohydrate________________grams

Protein_____________________grams

Fat_________________________grams

Calories____________________

INSULIN PRESCRIPTION:

Kind____________________________Number of Units______________

AND/OR
ORAL HYPOGLYCEMIC AGENT:

Kind____________________________ Dosage ______________________

OTHER MEDICATION:

AFFILIATES

of the American Diabetes Association

The American Diabetes Association has a number of Affiliate Associations, many of which have active lay groups, and others are in the process of formation. Information in regard to Affiliate Associations in specific areas may be secured from the American Diabetes Association, 18 East 48th Street, New York, New York 10017.

INDEX